Assessing Pain and Communication in Disorders of Consciousness

Recent advances in medicine for resuscitation and care have led to an increased number of patients who survive severe brain damage but who are poorly responsive and non-communicative at the bedside. This has led to a striking need to better characterize, understand and manage this population who present a real challenge for the assessment of pain and for planning treatment. This edited collection provides clinicians with a guide to recent developments in research on pain perception and assessment, and the detection of consciousness and communication in patients with disorders of consciousness (DOC).

With contributions from leading global researchers, the book gives an overview of issues concerning the assessment of pain. It also covers the development of suitable tools both to improve pain management and to detect consciousness and communication in these patients, in order to influence their prognosis and treatment and enhance their quality of life. Methodological and ethical issues relating to the implications for future research are also considered.

The book will be an invaluable guide for clinicians, medics, and therapists working in rehabilitation and acute care, particularly in the demanding field of pain perception, pain assessment, and detection of consciousness and communication in patients with DOC. It will also be useful for students and researchers in neuropsychology and the medical sciences.

Camille Chatelle is a postdoctoral research fellow at the Spaulding Rehabilitation Hospital Neurorehabilitation Laboratory, Harvard Medical School, USA. She is also working as a postdoctoral researcher at the Laboratory for Neuro-Imaging of Coma and Consciousness, Massachusetts General Hospital, Harvard Medical School, USA.

Steven Laureys leads the Coma Science Group at the Cyclotron Research Center and Department of Neurology, Sart Tilman Liège University Hospital, Belgium. He is Clinical Professor and Research Director at the Belgian National Fund of Scientific Research (FNRS).

Assessing Pain and Communication in Disorders of Consciousness

Edited by Camille Chatelle
and Steven Laureys

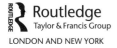

Routledge
Taylor & Francis Group

LONDON AND NEW YORK

First published 2016
by Routledge
2 Park Square, Milton Park, Abingdon, Oxon, OX14 4RN

and by Routledge
711 Third Avenue, New York, NY 10017

Routledge is an imprint of the Taylor & Francis Group, an informa business

© 2016 Camille Chatelle and Steven Laureys

British Library Cataloguing in Publication Data

A catalogue record for this book is available from the British Library

Library of Congress Cataloging-in-Publication Data
    Assessing pain and communication in disorders of consciousness / edited by Camille Chatelle and Steven Laureys.
        pages cm
    Includes bibliographical references and index.
    1. Brain damage—Imaging.   2. Loss of consciousness—Imaging.   3. Pain—Measurement.   4. Interpersonal communication—Testing.   I. Chatelle, Camille.   II. Laureys, Steven.
    RC387.5.A84 2016
    616.85'889—dc23
    2015021516

ISBN: 978-1-138-81480-6 (hbk)
ISBN: 978-1-138-81482-0 (pbk)
ISBN: 978-1-315-74720-0 (ebk)

Typeset in Bembo
by Apex CoVantage, LLC

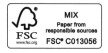

Printed and bound in Great Britain by
TJ International Ltd, Padstow, Cornwall

Contents

Colour Plates follow page 88

Series preface

Rehabilitation is a process whereby people who have been disabled by injury or illness work together with health service staff and others to achieve their optimum level of physical, psychological, social, and vocational well-being (McLellan, 1991). It includes all measures aimed at reducing the impact of handicapping and disabling conditions and at enabling disabled people to return to their most appropriate environment (Wilson, 1997; World Health Organization, 1986). Rehabilitation also includes attempts to alter impairment in underlying cognitive and brain systems by the provision of systematic, planned experience to the damaged brain (Robertson & Murre, 1999). All of this applies also to neuropsychological rehabilitation, which is concerned with the assessment, treatment, and natural recovery of people who have sustained an insult to the brain.

Neuropsychological rehabilitation is influenced by a number of fields both within and without psychology. Neuropsychology, behavioural psychology, and cognitive psychology have all played important roles in the development of current rehabilitation practice, as have findings from studies in neuroplasticity, linguistics, geriatric medicine, neurology, and other fields. Our discipline, therefore, is not confined to one conceptual framework; rather, it has a broad theoretical base.

We hope that this broad base is reflected in the modular handbooks in this series. The first book, by Roger Barker and Stephen Dunnett, set the scene by talking about *Neural repair, transplantation and rehabilitation*. The second title, by Josef Zihl, addressed visual disorders after brain injury. Other titles in the series include *Behavioural approaches in neuropsychological rehabilitation* by Barbara A. Wilson, Camilla Herbert, and Agnes Shiel; *Neuropsychological rehabilitation and people with dementia* by Linda Clare; and a second edition of Josef Zihl's book *Rehabilitation of visual disorders after brain injury*. The latest book is Tamara Ownsworth's *Self-identity after brain injury*, which covers a popular topic in current neuropsychological rehabilitation.

Future titles will include volumes on specific cognitive functions such as language, memory, and motor skills, together with social and personality aspects of neuropsychological rehabilitation, as this is the kind of handbook that can be added to over the years.

Although each volume will be based on a strong theoretical foundation relevant to the topic in question, the main thrust of the majority of the books will be the development of practical, clinical methods of rehabilitation arising out of this research enterprise.

The series is aimed at neuropsychologists, clinical psychologists, and other rehabilitation specialists such as occupational therapists, speech and language pathologists, rehabilitation physicians, and those working in other disciplines involved in the rehabilitation of people with brain injury.

Neuropsychological rehabilitation is at an exciting stage in its development. On the one hand, we have a huge growth of interest in functional imaging techniques that tell us about the basic processes going on in the brain. On the other hand, the past few years have seen the introduction of a number of theoretically driven approaches to cognitive rehabilitation from the fields of language, memory, attention, and perception. There is also a growing recognition among health-service professionals that rehabilitation is an integral part of a health-care system. Of course, alongside the recognition of the need for rehabilitation is the awareness that any system has to be evaluated. Among those of us working with brain-injured people, including patients with dementia, there is a feeling that things are moving forward. This series, we hope, is one reflection of this movement toward the integration of theory and practice.

Barbara A. Wilson

Ian H. Robertson

References

McLellan, D. L. (1991). Functional recovery and the principles of disability medicine. In M. Swash & J. Oxbury (Eds.), *Clinical neurology*. Edinburgh: Churchill Livingstone.

Robertson, I. H., & Murre, J. M. J. (1999). Rehabilitation of brain damage: Brain plasticity and principles of guided recovery. *Psychological Bulletin, 125*, 544–575.

Wilson, B. A. (1997). Cognitive rehabilitation: How it is and how it might be. *Journal of the International Neuropsychological Society, 3*, 487–496.

World Health Organization. (1986). *Optimum care of disabled people* (report of a WHO meeting). Turku, Finland: WHO.

1 Introduction to the challenge of pain and communication in disorders of consciousness

Camille Chatelle,[1] Steven Laureys,[2] and Caroline Schnakers[3]

Abbreviations

BCI	brain–computer interface
CRS-R	Coma Recovery Scale-Revised
DOC	disorders of consciousness
EEG	electroencephalography
fMRI	functional magnetic resonance imagery
LIS	locked-in syndrome
MCS	minimally conscious state
MCS+	minimally conscious state plus
MCS–	minimally conscious state minus
PET	positron emission tomography
VS/UWS	vegetative state/unresponsive wakefulness syndrome

Advances in medicine for resuscitation and care have led to an increased number of patients surviving severe brain damage. Some of them will quickly recover consciousness and will be able to communicate, while others may evolve into various disorders of consciousness (DOC). In this introductory chapter, we will define the different DOC that can follow a severe brain injury and the clinical challenges associated with these patients in terms of pain management and detection of consciousness and communication.

Behavioral definition of DOC following a severe brain injury

Although no commonly shared definition of consciousness exists, it is widely accepted that it is a multicomponent term involving a series of cognitive processes such as attention and memory (Baars, Ramsey, & Laureys, 2003; Zeman, 2005). It has been suggested that consciousness is underlined by a large frontoparietal network, also called the global neuronal workspace (Baars, 2005; Dehaene & Changeux, 2011). Additionally, neuroimaging studies have highlighted the importance of the thalamo-cortical connections, especially in the emergence of consciousness (Tononi & Koch, 2008). Indeed, in patients who have recovered consciousness, a reestablishment of the correlation between associative cortices and the thalamus has been observed (Laureys et al., 2000b).

At the bedside, consciousness can be characterized by two main components: arousal and awareness (Laureys, Faymonville, & Maquet, 2002a; Posner, Saper, Schiff, & Plum, 2007). Clinically, arousal is manifested by spontaneous eye opening, whereas awareness is assessed by responses to external stimuli (e.g., command-following, visual pursuit, adequate emotional response). Although loss of arousal is associated with altered awareness (e.g., sleep, anesthesia), preserved arousal level does not necessarily imply preserved awareness. Following severe brain damage, a patient can either die (brain death) or evolve through different states of altered consciousness before possibly recovering full consciousness. Each of these states is associated with more or less severe cognitive and motor disabilities (see Figure 1.1). As shown in Figure 1.1, the restoration of spontaneous or elicited eye opening, in the absence of voluntary motor activity, marks the transition from coma to vegetative state/unresponsive wakefulness syndrome (VS/UWS). The passage from VS/UWS to the minimally conscious state minus (MCS−) is marked by the appearance of non-linguistic signs of conscious awareness. MCS plus (MCS+) patients show clear evidence of receptive or expressive language function. Emergence from MCS is signaled by the return of functional communication or object use. The locked-in syndrome (LIS) is the extreme example of intact cognition with nearly complete or complete motor

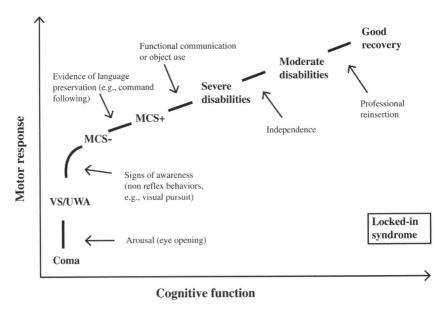

Figure 1.1 Different clinical entities encountered on the gradual recovery from coma, illustrated as a function of cognitive and motor ability (adapted from Chatelle & Laureys, 2011).

deficit (Laureys, Perrin, Schnakers, Boly, & Majerus, 2005b). Each of these states has also been studied in terms of brain metabolism at rest or brain activation in response to external stimuli.

Brain death

The term "brain death" suggests that the organism cannot function as a whole. Critical functions such as respiration, blood pressure, neuroendocrine and homeostatic regulation, and consciousness are permanently lacking. The patient is apneic and unreactive to environmental stimulation (Guidelines for the determination of death, 1981). This term can only be used after bedside demonstration of irreversible cessation of functions of the brain and the brainstem. Brain death is usually caused by a severe brain lesion (e.g., massive traumatic injury, intracranial hemorrhage, or anoxia) resulting in an intracranial pressure higher than the mean arterial blood pressure. The diagnosis can be made within 6–24 hours, after excluding pharmacological or toxic treatments or hypothermia as potential confounders. This state is characterized by the absence of residual brain metabolism, confirming the absence of neuronal function in the whole brain (Laureys, Owen, & Schiff, 2004a).

Coma

Some patients can remain in a coma, neither aroused nor aware, for several weeks. Their eyes are constantly closed and they do not manifest voluntary behavioral responses. Generally, patients emerge from their comatose state within two to four weeks (Posner et al., 2007). The prognosis is influenced by different factors such as etiology, the patient's general medical condition, and age. Outcome is most likely to be bad if, after three days of observation, there are still no pupillary or corneal reflexes, there is stereotyped or no motor responses to noxious stimulation, and an isoelectrical or burst-suppression electrophysiological (EEG) pattern is observed. Prognosis in traumatic coma survivors is better than in anoxic cases (Whyte et al., 2009). Recovery from coma may lead to a vegetative state, a minimally conscious state or, more rarely, to a locked-in syndrome (Bruno, Vanhaudenhuyse, Thibaut, Moonen, & Laureys, 2011; Posner et al., 2007). Coma is generally associated with a global decrease in brain metabolism of 50–70% of the normal range.

Vegetative state/unresponsive wakefulness syndrome

The "vegetative state" (VS), "an organic body capable of growth and development but devoid of sensation and thought," was defined in 1972 by Jennett and Plum (Jennett & Plum, 1972). The term was proposed to describe a state in which autonomic functions (e.g., cardio-vascular regulation, thermoregulation) and arousal (wakefulness and rest cycles) were preserved with the absence of awareness. Behaviorally, patients in VS open their eyes spontaneously or in response to stimulation, but they only show reflexive (involuntary) responses to the environment. Recently, some have suggested replacing the term VS with "unresponsive wakefulness syndrome" (UWS) in order to avoid the negative association with the word "vegetative" and to better describe the behavioral pattern observed in this population (Laureys et al., 2010). It has been suggested that the state can be defined as permanent when there is no recovery after a specified period (three or twelve months, depending on etiology, anoxic or traumatic, respectively) (American Congress of Rehabilitation Medicine, 1995; Jennett, 2005). However, further evidence suggests that patients in a VS/UWS can recover even after this length of time, so the term may therefore not be appropriate (Estraneo et al., 2013; Estraneo, Moretta, Loreto, Santoro, & Trojano, 2014). Studies on global brain metabolism have usually shown a decrease of about 40–50% of normal range values in VS/UWS patients (Stender et al., 2015), although some studies have reported cerebral metabolism (Schiff et al., 2002) or blood flow (Agardh, Rosen, & Ryding, 1983) in the normal range in some cases.

Minimally conscious state

Patients in a minimally conscious state (MCS) are aroused and manifest fluctuating but consistent and reproducible signs of awareness (Giacino et al., 2002). Visual pursuit appears to be an early behavioral marker of the transition from VS/UWS to MCS (Giacino & Whyte, 2005), but these patients can also show other voluntary behavioral responses and/or oriented emotional reactions such as responses to verbal orders, object manipulation, oriented responses to noxious stimulation, visual fixation, or appropriate crying/smiling. However, responsiveness can fluctuate, which makes the detection of voluntary behaviors at the bedside challenging. Some researchers have recently proposed subcategorizing MCS into MCS minus (MCS−) and MCS plus (MCS+), based on evidence of differences in brain metabolism within the language network (Bruno et al., 2012; Bruno et al., 2011). MCS+ would encompass patients who show clear evidence of receptive or expressive language function (e.g., command-following). In contrast, MCS− would define those who demonstrate only nonlinguistic signs of conscious awareness (e.g., visual pursuit). The specific behaviors required to meet the criteria for MCS+ and MCS− are still being discussed and additional empirical investigation is needed before these categories can be implemented in clinical practice.

Emergence from MCS is defined by the recovery of functional communication and/or functional use of objects (Giacino et al., 2002). Some patients can remain in MCS without fully recovering consciousness for a prolonged period (Fins, Schiff, & Foley, 2007). Prognosis for recovery in MCS patients remains very difficult because of the marked heterogeneity in the underlying pathophysiology of these patients. However, a better outcome for MCS as compared to VS/UWS patients has been reported (Lammi, Smith, Tate, & Taylor, 2005; Luauté et al., 2010). If the global metabolic rate remains usually higher in MCS than in VS/UWS (Stender et al., 2015), it does not always show substantial changes and return to normal after recovery of consciousness (Laureys, Lemaire, Maquet, Phillips, & Franck, 1999). However, activation studies reported differences between MCS and VS/UWS patients, suggesting a disparity between cognitive preservation and processing of external stimuli such as pain (see also Chapter 2 and 3).

Locked-in syndrome

Not to be misidentified as patients suffering from an altered state of consciousness, locked-in (LIS) patients cannot move or talk but they are usually able to use vertical eye movements and/or blink to communicate. This syndrome is often due to a selective supranuclear motor deefferentation that results in the paralysis of all four limbs and the last cranial nerves without interfering with consciousness (American Congress of Rehabilitation Medicine, 1995; Plum & Posner, 1983) or cognition (Schnakers et al., 2008b). Therefore, these patients may present the same behavioral pattern as that observed in VS/UWS or MCS patients, which often leads to misdiagnosis of altered state of consciousness (see also Chapter 8). LIS can be subcategorized based on the extent of motor impairment (Bauer, Gerstenbrand, & Rumpl, 1979): patients with classical LIS are totally immobile but can make vertical eye movements and blink; incomplete LIS is characterized by remnant nonocular voluntary motions (e.g., head or finger movements); and total LIS patients are completely paralyzed and have no eye movement (see also Chapter 6). When looking at the brain metabolism of these patients, researchers observed no significant decrease in metabolism in the supratentorial gray matter as compared with healthy subjects (Laureys et al., 2005a). However, a positron emission tomography (PET) study by Levy et al. reported a 25% reduction in cerebral metabolism in three LIS patients as compared to healthy controls (Levy et al., 1987).

Cortical processing in disorders of consciousness

Several neuroimaging studies using PET and functional magnetic resonance imagery (fMRI) have studied brain processing in response to stimulation in patients with DOC. Following auditory and nociceptive stimulation, limited brain activation was reported in a majority of VS/UWS patients, whereas MCS patients showed an activity level close to that observed in control subjects (Boly et al., 2005; Boly et al., 2008; Laureys et al., 2000a). More specifically, activation studies performed on a VS/UWS group using auditory stimulation (i.e., tones) showed preserved functioning of the primary auditory cortex but without involvement of other brain areas (such as the temporoparietal junction; Laureys et al., 2000a). Following noxious stimulation (i.e., electrical stimulation of the median nerve), an increase in activity could be observed in the midbrain, contralateral thalamus, and primary somatosensory cortex, but again with limited activation in higher-order brain areas more deeply involved in perception processing (Kassubek et al., 2003; Kotchoubey et al., 2013; Laureys et al., 2002b;

Markl et al., 2013; see also Chapter 2). Additionally, low-order primary cortical activity seemed to be isolated from higher-order associative cortical activity in VS/UWS patients (Laureys et al., 2002b). On the other hand, auditory and nociceptive stimulations of MCS patients led to widespread activation involving associative cortices considered hierarchically superior in the processing of sensory information. Such activation suggests that these patients have partially preserved auditory and pain processing (Boly et al., 2005; Boly et al., 2008; Laureys et al., 2000a; Schiff et al., 2005). Other studies have also reported widespread activation in the temporal, insular, and amygdala areas in response to stimuli with emotional valence (Bekinschtein et al., 2004; Laureys et al., 2004b).

Clinical diagnosis: pain and communication

While neuroimaging studies offer a great means to better understand brain processing in DOC, the majority of the findings is based on group analyses and can be difficult to apply to individual patients in clinical settings. Additionally, it remains difficult to interpret the significance of partially or fully preserved brain activation in terms of a patient's conscious awareness of the self and the environment and his or her subjective experience.

In terms of pain management in patients with DOC, the assessment is limited by the difficulty or impossibility of establishing functional communication. The inability of the patient to provide a subjective report leads to potential ethical and medical concerns. In both acute and chronic stages, several conditions – such as polytraumatic injuries, open wounds, and spasticity – are likely to induce pain, especially during care and mobilization (Chatelle et al., 2014). The need for analgesic treatment and close monitoring is therefore evident, and especially in light of previous studies suggesting pain perception capacity in patients with DOC. A European survey asked over 2,000 medical and paramedical professionals about their beliefs regarding possible pain perception in patients with DOC. Their answers regarding whether or not these patients (VS/UWS or MCS) can feel pain were very different. Interestingly, the opinions of these healthcare professionals varied according to their profession, religious beliefs, and region of origin (Demertzi et al., 2009). The disparity in opinions and perceptions of pain among caregivers may lead to variability in pain and symptom management. Given the challenges of defining levels of consciousness in this population (Schnakers et al., 2009) and considering the degree of clinical uncertainty regarding pain perception, pain treatment should be considered for all patients (Chatelle et al., 2012; Monti et al., 2010; Schnakers et al., 2009) and should be managed using standardized procedures (i.e., behavioral scales) (Chatelle et al., 2014; see also Chapters 3 and 4). However, until now no clear guidelines for pain management in cases of DOC have been proposed.

In the context of pain assessment, obtaining an accurate diagnosis of the patient's level of consciousness and communication is really important. The patient's quality of life and outcome may depend on an accurate assessment at the bedside. In addition to differences in brain processing in VS/UWS and MCS patients, outcome studies have reported that MCS patients usually have a better prognosis than those with VS/UWS (Katz, Polyak, Coughlan, Nichols, & Roche, 2009; Luauté et al., 2010). In addition, some patients might be diagnosed as VS/UWS or MCS despite their suffering from LIS (see Chapter 6) and therefore processing fully painful conditions.

Currently, the clinical diagnosis of consciousness is mainly based on behavioral assessment at the bedside. The detection of oriented/voluntary responses and functional communication is really important for detecting consciousness as both signs of response and communication, respectively, indicate emergence from VS/UWS and MCS. Functional communication also differentiates LIS from VS/UWS patients. However, the difficulty of objectively distinguishing reflexive from voluntary responses makes the assessment very challenging for clinicians.

In this context, the use of standardized tools can help the examiner to limit errors associated with subjectivity (see Chapter 3). Schnakers et al. (2009) reported that 41% of patients were diagnosed incorrectly by expert team consensus, when compared to the diagnoses obtained using a standardized assessment instrument, the Coma Recovery Scale-Revised (CRS-R) (Giacino, Kalmar, & Whyte, 2004). This data suggests that the use of a sensitive scale is crucial when assessing consciousness (Schnakers et al., 2008a).

On the other hand, standardized behavioral assessments are complicated by motor disabilities, aphasia (Majerus, Bruno, Schnakers, Giacino, & Laureys, 2009), fluctuation in arousal level and vigilance (Giacino et al., 2002), and other physical impairments such as blindness or deafness. Because of these compromising factors, it can be very difficult to make an accurate diagnosis. It is therefore important to develop other paraclinical tools to detect signs of consciousness and communication when no response can be observed at the bedside. As misdiagnosis can lead to grave ethical consequences, especially in terms of end-of-life decision-making (Andrews, 2004) and pain treatment (Chatelle et al., 2014), additional tools should be used to assess remnant cognitive abilities in patients with DOC.

In this context, new technologies such as electroencephalography, PET, or fMRI could provide paraclinical tools that bypass the motor pathway and allow clinicians to detect consciousness. In the last decade, studies have reported the potential of these techniques to probe command-following in severely brain-injured patients by asking them to actively modulate their brain activity during a specific task (Chatelle et al., 2012; Chatelle, Lesenfants, Guller, Laureys, & Noirhomme, 2015). By extension, these methods could be used to control a brain-computer interface (BCI). BCI, by definition, uses brain activity alone to drive external devices or computer interfaces (Wolpaw, Birbaumer, McFarland, Pfurtscheller, & Vaughan, 2002). Recent studies have shown the usefulness of BCIs in controlling motor prostheses, cursors, access to the Internet, and communication (Citi, Poli, Cinel, & Sepulveda, 2008; Lee, Ryu, Jolesz, Cho, & Yoo, 2009; Mugler, Ruf, Halder, Bensch, & Kler, 2010; Müller-Putz & Pfurtscheller, 2008; Sellers, Vaughan, & Wolpaw, 2010; Yoo et al., 2004). In this context, the development of accurate BCIs enabling command-following or even a simple binary communication code would have a huge impact, from a clinical perspective as well as from a social one (see Chapter 5). BCI may make it possible for some behaviorally noncommunicative patients to participate in their treatment, to tell their caregivers/family how they feel and when/where they are in pain, and also to report about their desire to live or to die. However, the introduction of these technologies in clinical settings will also raise important ethical discussions (see Chapter 7).

In this book, we aim to provide clinicians with the most up-to-date information in the field of clinical diagnosis of pain and communication in DOC, including ethical reflections and evidence-based recommendations for managing care in this population.

Notes

1 **Camille Chatelle** is a postdoctoral research fellow at the Neurorehabilitation Lab at the Spaulding Rehabilitation Hospital, Harvard Medical School. She is also working as a postdoctoral researcher at the Laboratory for NeuroImaging of Coma and Consciousness at Massachusetts General Hospital, Harvard Medical School.
2 **Steven Laureys** leads the Coma Science Group at the Cyclotron Research Center and Department of Neurology, Sart Tilman Liège University Hospital, Belgium. He is Clinical Professor and Research Director at the Belgian National Fund of Scientific Research (FNRS).
3 **Caroline Schnakers**, PhD, Department of Neurosurgery University of California–Los Angeles Los Angeles, CA, USA.

References

Agardh, C. D., Rosen, I., & Ryding, E. (1983). Persistent vegetative state with high cerebral blood flow following profound hypoglycemia. *Ann Neurol, 14*(4), 482–486.

American Congress of Rehabilitation Medicine. (1995). Recommendations for use of uniform nomenclature pertinent to patients with severe alterations in consciousness. *Arch Phys Med Rehabil, 76*(2), 205–209.

Andrews, K. (2004). Medical decision making in the vegetative state: withdrawal of nutrition and hydration. *NeuroRehabilitation, 19*(4), 299–304.

Baars, B. J. (2005). Global workspace theory of consciousness: toward a cognitive neuroscience of human experience. *Prog Brain Res, 150*, 45–53.

Baars, B. J., Ramsey, T. Z., & Laureys, S. (2003). Brain, conscious experience and the observing self. *Trends in Neuroscience, 26*(12), 671–675.

Bauer, G., Gerstenbrand, F., & Rumpl, E. (1979). Varieties of the locked-in syndrome. *J Neurol, 221*, 77–91.

Bekinschtein, T., Leiguarda, R., Armony, J., Owen, A., Carpintiero, S., Niklison, J., . . . Manes, F. (2004). Emotion processing in the minimally conscious state. *J Neurol Neurosurg Psychiatry, 75*(5), 788.

Boly, M., Faymonville, M. E., Peigneux, P., Lambermont, B., Damas, F., Luxen, A., . . . Laureys, S. (2005). Cerebral processing of auditory and noxious stimuli in severely brain injured patients: differences between VS and MCS. *Neuropsychological Rehabilitation, 15*(3/4), 283–289.

Boly, M., Faymonville, M. E., Schnakers, C., Peigneux, P., Lambermont, B., Phillips, C., . . . Laureys, S. (2008). Perception of pain in the minimally conscious state with PET activation: an observational study. *The Lancet Neurology, 7*(11), 1013–1020.

Bruno, M. A., Majerus, S., Boly, M., Vanhaudenhuyse, A., Schnakers, C., Gosseries, O., . . . Laureys, S. (2012). Functional neuroanatomy underlying the clinical subcategorization of minimally conscious state patients. *J Neurol, 259*(6):1087–1098.

Bruno, M. A., Vanhaudenhuyse, A., Thibaut, A., Moonen, G., & Laureys, S. (2011). From unresponsive wakefulness to minimally conscious PLUS and functional locked-in syndromes: recent advances in our understanding of disorders of consciousness. *J Neurol, 258*(7), 1373–1384.

Chatelle, C., Chennu, S., Noirhomme, Q., Cruse, D., Owen, A. M., & Laureys, S. (2012). Brain-computer interfacing in disorders of consciousness. *Brain Inj, 26*(12), 1510–1522.

Chatelle, C., & Laureys, S. (2011). Understanding disorders of consciousness. In J. Illes and B. J. Sahakian (Eds.), *The Oxford Handbook of Neuroethics* (pp. 119–133). New York: Oxford University Press.

Chatelle, C., Lesenfants, D., Guller, Y., Laureys, S., & Noirhomme, Q. (2015). Brain-computer interface for assessing consciousness in severely brain-injured patients. In A. Rossetti & S. Laureys (Eds.), *Clinical Neurophysiology in Disorders of Consciousness* (pp. 133–148). Wien: Springer-Verlag.

Chatelle, C., Thibaut, A., Whyte, J., De Val, M. D., Laureys, S., & Schnakers, C. (2014). Pain issues in disorders of consciousness. *Brain Inj, 28*(9), 1202–1208.

Citi, L., Poli, R., Cinel, C., & Sepulveda, F. (2008). P300-based BCI mouse with genetically-optimized analogue control. *IEEE Trans Neural Syst Rehabil Eng, 16*(1), 51–61.

Dehaene, S., & Changeux, J. P. (2011). Experimental and theoretical approaches to conscious processing. *Neuron, 70*(2), 200–227.

Demertzi, A., Schnakers, C., Ledoux, D., Chatelle, C., Bruno, M. A., Vanhaudenhuyse, A., . . . Laureys, S. (2009). Different beliefs about pain perception in the vegetative and minimally conscious states: a European survey of medical and paramedical professionals. *Prog Brain Res, 177*, 329–338.

Estraneo, A., Moretta, P., Loreto, V., Lanzillo, B., Cozzolino, A., Saltalamacchia, A., . . . Trojano, L. (2013). Predictors of recovery of responsiveness in prolonged anoxic vegetative state. *Neurology, 80*(5), 464–470.

Estraneo, A., Moretta, P., Loreto, V., Santoro, L., & Trojano, L. (2014). Clinical and neuropsychological long-term outcomes after late recovery of responsiveness: a case series. *Arch Phys Med Rehabil, 95*(4), 711–716.

Fins, J. J., Schiff, N. D., & Foley, K. M. (2007). Late recovery from the minimally conscious state: ethical and policy implications. *Neurology, 68*(4), 304–307.

Giacino, J., Ashwal, S., Childs, N., Cranford, R., Jennett, B., Katz, D., . . . Zafonte, R. (2002). The minimally conscious state: definition and diagnostic criteria. *Neurology, 58*(3), 349–353.

Giacino, J., Kalmar, K., & Whyte, J. (2004). The JFK Coma Recovery Scale-Revised: measurement characteristics and diagnostic utility. *Arch Phys Med Rehabil, 85*(12), 2020–2029.

Giacino, J., & Whyte, J. (2005). The vegetative and minimally conscious states: current knowledge and remaining questions. *J Head Trauma Rehabil, 20*(1), 30–50.

Guidelines for the determination of death. (1981). Report of the medical consultants on the diagnosis of death to the President's Commission for the Study of Ethical Problems in Medicine and Biomedical and Behavioral Research. *JAMA, 246*(19), 2184–2186.

Jennett, B. (2005). Thirty years of the vegetative state: clinical, ethical and legal problems. In S. Laureys (Ed.), *The Boundaries of Consciousness: Neurobiology and Neuropathology, 150* (pp. 537–543). Amsterdam: Elsevier.

Jennett, B., & Plum, F. (1972). Persistent vegetative state after brain damage: a syndrome in search of a name. *Lancet, 1*, 734–737.

Kassubek, J., Juengling, F. D., Els, T., Spreer, J., Herpers, M., Krause, T., . . . Lücking, C. H. (2003). Activation of a residual cortical network during painful stimulation in long-term postanoxic vegetative state: a ^{15}O–H$_2$O PET study. *J Neurological Sciences, 212*, 85–91.

Katz, D. I., Polyak, M., Coughlan, D., Nichols, M., & Roche, A. (2009). Natural history of recovery from brain injury after prolonged disorders of consciousness: outcome of patients admitted to inpatient rehabilitation with 1–4 year follow-up. *Prog Brain Res, 177*, 73–88.

Kotchoubey, B., Merz, S., Lang, S., Markl, A., Muller, F., Yu, T., & Schwarzbauer, C. (2013). Global functional connectivity reveals highly significant differences between the vegetative and the minimally conscious state. *J Neurol, 260*(4), 975–983.

Lammi, M. H., Smith, V. H., Tate, R. L., & Taylor, C. M. (2005). The minimally conscious state and recovery potential: a follow-up study 2 to 5 years after traumatic brain injury. *Arch Phys Med Rehabil, 86*(4), 746–754.

Laureys, S., Celesia, G. G., Cohadon, F., Lavrijsen, J., Leon-Carrion, J., Sannita, W. G., . . . Dolce, G. (2010). Unresponsive wakefulness syndrome: a new name for the vegetative state or apallic syndrome. *BMC Med, 8*, 68.

Laureys, S., Faymonville, M. E., Degueldre, C., Fiore, G. D., Damas, P., Lambermont, B., et al. (2000a). Auditory processing in the vegetative state. *Brain, 123*, 1589–1601.

Laureys, S., Faymonville, M. E., Luxen, A., Lamy, M., Franck, G., & Maquet, P. (2000b). Restoration of thalamocortical connectivity after recovery from persistent vegetative state. *The Lancet, 355*(9217), 1790–1791.

Laureys, S., Faymonville, M., & Maquet, P. (2002a). Quelle conscience durant le coma? *Pour la science, 302*, 122–128.

Laureys, S., Faymonville, M., Peigneux, P., Damas, P., Lambermont, B., Del Fiore, G., . . . Franck, G. (2002b). Cortical processing of noxious somatosensory stimuli in the persistent vegetative state. *Neuroimage, 17*(2), 732–741.

Laureys, S., Lemaire, C., Maquet, P., Phillips, C., & Franck, G. (1999). Cerebral metabolism during vegetative state and after recovery to consciousness. *J Neurol, Neurosurg & Psychiatry, 67*, 121.

Laureys, S., Owen, A., & Schiff, D. (2004a). Brain function in coma, vegetative state and related disorders. *The Lancet Neurology, 3*, 537–546.

Laureys, S., Pellas, F., Van Eeckhout, P., Ghorbel, S., Schnakers, C., Perrin, F., . . . Goldman, S. (2005a). The locked-in syndrome: what is it like to be conscious but paralyzed and voiceless? *Prog Brain Res, 150*, 495–511.

Laureys, S., Perrin, F., Faymonville, M., Schnakers, C., Boly, M., Bartsch, V., . . . Maquet, P. (2004b). Cerebral processing in the minimally conscious state. *Neurology, 63*, 916–918.

Laureys, S., Perrin, F., Schnakers, C., Boly, M., & Majerus, S. (2005b). Residual cognitive function in comatose, vegetative and minimally conscious states. *Current opinion in neurology, 18*, 726–733.

Lee, J. H., Ryu, J., Jolesz, F. A., Cho, Z. H., & Yoo, S. S. (2009). Brain-machine interface via real-time fMRI: preliminary study on thought-controlled robotic arm. *Neurosci Lett, 450*(1), 1–6.

Levy, D. E., Sidtis, J. J., Rottenberg, D. A., Jarden, J. O., Strother, S. C., Dhawan, V., . . . Plum, F. (1987). Differences in cerebral blood flow and glucose utilization in vegetative versus locked-in patients. *Ann Neurol, 22*(6), 673–682.

Luauté, J., Maucort-Boulch, D., Tell, L., Quelard, F., Sarraf, T., Iwaz, J., . . . Fischer, C. (2010). Long-term outcomes of chronic minimally conscious and vegetative states. *Neurology, 75*(3), 246–252.

Majerus, S., Bruno, M. A., Schnakers, C., Giacino, J. T., & Laureys, S. (2009). The problem of aphasia in the assessment of consciousness in brain-damaged patients. *Prog Brain Res, 177,* 49–61.

Markl, A., Yu, T., Vogel, D., Muller, F., Kotchoubey, B., & Lang, S. (2013). Brain processing of pain in patients with unresponsive wakefulness syndrome. *Brain Behav, 3*(2), 95–103.

Monti, M. M., Vanhaudenhuyse, A., Coleman, M. R., Boly, M., Pickard, J. D., Tshibanda, L., . . . Laureys, S. (2010). Willful modulation of brain activity in disorders of consciousness. *N Engl J Med, 362*(7), 579–589.

Mugler, E. M., Ruf, C. A., Halder, S., Bensch, M., & Kler, A. (2010). Design and implementation of a P300-based brain-computer interface for controlling an Internet browser. *IEEE Trans Neural Syst Rehabil Eng, 18*(6), 599–609.

Müller-Putz, G. R., & Pfurtscheller, G. (2008). Control of an electrical prosthesis with an SSVEP-based BCI. *IEEE Trans Biomed Eng, 55*(1), 361–364.

Plum, F., & Posner, J. B. (1983). *The diagnosis of stupor and coma* (3rd ed.). Philadelphia: FA Davis.

Posner, J., Saper, C., Schiff, N., & Plum, F. (2007). *Plum and Posner's diagnosis of stupor and coma.* New York: Oxford University Press.

Schiff, N. D., Ribary, U., Moreno, R., Beattie, B., Kronberg, E., Blasberg, R., . . . Plum, F. (2002). Residual cerebral activity and behavioural fragments can remain in the persistently vegetative brain. *Brain, 125*(6), 1210–1234.

Schiff, N. D., Rodriguez-Moreno, D., Kamal, A., Kim, K. H. S., Giacino, J. T., Plum, F., Hirsch, J. (2005). fMRI reveals large-scale network activation in minimally conscious patients. *Neurology, 64*(3), 514–523.

Schnakers, C., Majerus, S., Giacino, J., Vanhaudenhuyse, A., Bruno, M., Boly, M., . . . Lamy, M. (2008a). A French validation study of the Coma Recovery Scale-Revised (CRS-R). *Brain Injury, 22*(10), 786–792.

Schnakers, C., Majerus, S., Goldman, S., Boly, M., Van Eeckhout, P., Gay, S., . . . Laureys, S. (2008b). Cognitive function in the locked-in syndrome. *J Neurol, 255*(3), 323–330.

Schnakers, C., Vanhaudenhuyse, A., Giacino, J., Ventura, M., Boly, M., Majerus, S., . . . Laureys, S. (2009). Diagnostic accuracy of the vegetative and minimally conscious state: clinical consensus versus standardized neurobehavioral assessment. *BMC Neurology, 9*(1), 35.

Sellers, E. W., Vaughan, T. M., & Wolpaw, J. R. (2010). A brain-computer interface for long-term independent home use. *Amyotroph Lateral Scler, 11*(5), 449–455.

Stender, J., Kupers, R., Rodell, A., Thibaut, A., Chatelle, C., Bruno, M. A., . . . Gjedde, A. (2015). Quantitative rates of brain glucose metabolism distinguish minimally conscious from vegetative state patients. *J Cereb Blood Flow Metab, 35*(1), 58–65.

Tononi, G., & Koch, C. (2008). The neural correlates of consciousness: an update. *Ann N Y Acad Sci, 1124,* 239–261.

Whyte, J., Gosseries, O., Chervoneva, I., DiPasquale, M. C., Giacino, J., Kalmar, K., . . . Eifert, B. (2009). Predictors of short-term outcome in brain-injured patients with disorders of consciousness. *Prog Brain Res, 177,* 63–72.

Wolpaw, J. R., Birbaumer, N., McFarland, D. J., Pfurtscheller, G., & Vaughan, T. M. (2002). Brain-computer interfaces for communication and control. *Clin Neurophysiol, 113*(6), 767–791.

Yoo, S. S., Fairreny, T., Chen, N. K., Choo, S. E., Panych, L. P., Park, H., . . . Jolesz, F. A. (2004). Brain-computer interface using fMRI: spatial navigation by thoughts. *Neuroreport, 15*(10), 1591–1595.

Zeman, A. (2005). What in the world is consciousness? *Prog Brain Res, 150,* 1–10.

2 The cortical processing of pain

André Mouraux[1]

Abbreviations

ACC	anterior cingulate cortex
BOLD	blood oxygen level-dependent
EEG	electroencephalography
ERP	event-related potential
ERF	event-related magnetic field
fMRI	functional magnetic resonance imaging
GBO	gamma-band oscillations
LFP	local field potential
MCS	minimally conscious state
MEG	magnetoencephalography
MVPA	multivariate pattern analysis
PET	positron emission tomography
PVS	persistent vegetative state
rCBF	regional cerebral blood flow
SS-EP	steady-state evoked potential
S1	primary somatosensory cortex
S2	secondary somatosensory cortex

Introduction

The development of non-invasive functional neuroimaging techniques has prompted an unparalleled increase in studies investigating the neural basis of perception in humans. In the field of pain, a large number of studies using functional magnetic resonance imaging (fMRI), positron emission tomography (PET), magnetoencephalography (MEG), or electroencephalography (EEG) have shown that when a noxious sensory stimulus is applied to the human skin, it elicits neuronal activity within a vast network of brain regions, including the primary somatosensory cortex (S1), the secondary somatosensory cortex (S2), the insula, and the anterior portion of the cingulate cortex (ACC) (Apkarian, Bushnell, Treede, & Zubieta, 2005; Bushnell & Apkarian, 2006; Garcia-Larrea, Frot, & Valeriani, 2003; Peyron, Laurent, & Garcia-Larrea, 2000; Tracey & Mantyh, 2007).

Furthermore, it has been repeatedly shown that the magnitude of responses evoked by noxious stimuli in this network of brain regions correlates with the intensity of stimulus-evoked pain (Coghill, Sang, Maisog, & Iadarola, 1999; Porro, 2003; Rainville, 2002). Hence, it has been suggested that these brain responses could be used as a biomarker for the experience of pain, and that the magnitude of these brain responses could be used to assess the amount of pain perceived by a human subject (Miller, 2009; Schweinhardt, Bountra, & Tracey, 2006; Wager et al., 2013).

This suggestion raises an interesting possibility. Could the non-invasive methods used to sample brain activity be used to assess whether patients with disorders of consciousness have the ability to perceive pain? Furthermore, could these methods be used to assess whether or not, at a given moment in time, patients are experiencing pain?

The objective of the present chapter is to critically examine these possibilities, taking into consideration current knowledge of the functional significance of the brain activity related to pain in humans.

Cortical representation of transient exteroceptive pain

A great number of studies have characterized the brain responses elicited by the *transient activation of skin nociceptors* (Bushnell & Apkarian, 2006; Garcia-Larrea et al., 2003; Ingvar, 1999; Peyron et al., 2000; Porro, 2003; Tracey & Mantyh, 2007; Treede, Kenshalo, Gracely, & Jones, 1999). Nociceptors constitute a specific class of sensory receptors specifically devoted to the transduction of noxious sensory stimuli – that is, stimuli having the potential to inflict tissue damage (Sherrington, 1906). Nociceptors are not defined by the type of physical energy to which they respond but by their relatively elevated activation threshold. Indeed, nociceptors have the ability to transduce high-intensity mechanical or thermal stimuli, as well as some chemical stimuli. For this reason, nociception is sometimes considered to form a specific sensory modality, whose aim would be to signal potential threat to the body's integrity and trigger appropriate defensive reactions vital for survival (Legrain, Iannetti, Plaghki, & Mouraux, 2010).

Although the activation of peripheral nociceptors can produce pain, nociception is not synonymous with pain, which is a conscious experience. The activation of nociceptors can trigger reflex somatic and autonomic responses without necessarily generating a conscious experience of pain (Hofbauer, Fiset, Plourde, Backman, & Bushnell, 2004; Wall, McMahon, & Koltzenburg, 2006). Furthermore, pain can be perceived in the absence of nociception (Flor, Nikolajsen, & Staehelin Jensen, 2006). At present, it is generally agreed that pain originates from cortical processing (Treede et al., 1999). However, it is interesting to highlight that this notion is a relatively recent one. Indeed, Head and Holmes (1911) proposed that the perception of pain derives from thalamic, rather than cortical, activity.

After reviewing the different methods that can be used to generate transient pain in humans and describing the brain responses that can be sampled using non-invasive electrophysiological and functional neuroimaging techniques, we will assess whether these brain responses can be used to build models of how pain is represented in the human brain.

Experimental methods to generate transient exteroceptive pain in humans

To characterize the cortical processing of nociceptive input in humans requires a means to activate nociceptors in a selective fashion (Plaghki & Mouraux, 2003, 2005). If the stimulus also activates other types of sensory receptors, such as low-threshold mechanoreceptors, it becomes very difficult to distinguish between brain activity related to the processing of nociceptive input and brain activity related to the processing of non-nociceptive input.

Achieving this selective activation is technically challenging. For example, nociceptive afferents can be activated using transcutaneous electrical nerve stimulation. However, because the electrical activation threshold of large-diameter fibres is lower than that of small-diameter fibres, transcutaneous electrical stimulation of nociceptive fibres will also activate non-nociceptive afferents, particularly large-diameter A-beta fibres involved in the perception of touch.[2] Similarly, punctate mechanical probes can be used to activate mechanosensitive nociceptors and generate a clear perception of pinprick pain, but the probes are likely to also activate low-threshold mechanoreceptors.[3]

It is for these reasons that the majority of studies exploring the cortical representation of acute pain in humans has relied on thermal stimulation to selectively activate heat-sensitive nociceptors. Heating the skin will selectively activate heat-sensitive free nerve endings without concomitantly activating non-nociceptive fibres, thus generating an afferent volley that is entirely specific for the spinothalamic system. Several methods can be used to generate the thermal stimuli, such as contact thermodes and infrared lasers (Plaghki & Mouraux, 2003, 2005). One important advantage of infrared lasers is that the stimulus can be delivered without any skin contact and, hence, without any confound related to the activation of low-threshold mechanoreceptors (Carmon, Mor, & Goldberg, 1976; Plaghki & Mouraux, 2003, 2005).

Brain responses related to transient exteroceptive pain

The cortical responses to a transient exteroceptive nociceptive stimulus can be explored non-invasively using neuroimaging techniques providing in vivo information about brain function. This includes non-invasive electrophysiological techniques such as EEG and MEG that measure changes in scalp potential or magnetic fields related mainly to synchronized postsynaptic activity occurring in cortical pyramidal cells (Nunez & Srinivasan, 2006). Metabolic techniques can also be used, such as PET or fMRI performed using the blood oxygen level-dependent (BOLD) contrast to measure local changes in blood flow resulting from neurovascular coupling (Arthurs & Boniface, 2002; DiNuzzo, 2014).

Event-related potentials and event-related magnetic fields

The occurrence of a sensory, motor, or cognitive event can elicit transient changes in brain activity, some of which can be sampled using EEG or MEG (Box 1).

Box 1: Brain activity sampled using EEG and MEG

It is important to take into consideration the fact that only a fraction of stimulus-evoked changes in brain activity actually translates into a measurable EEG or MEG signal, because the activity must satisfy a number of conditions to be detected (Mouraux & Iannetti, 2008). First, it must generate a relatively strong electric or magnetic field and, therefore, must involve a relatively large population of neurons. Second, the activity elicited within each neuron of the activated population must be synchronous. If unitary activity is dispersed temporally, the resulting electric or magnetic fields will be spread over time and the related change in EEG or MEG signal will be difficult to measure. Third, the distance between the source of neuronal activity and the recording sensor must be small, as the amplitude of the signal measured at the sensors falls off rapidly with increased distance. The magnitude of the brain potentials or magnetic fields elicited by a given stimulus is often several factors smaller than the magnitude of the ongoing background activity. Therefore, researchers rely on signal-processing methods to enhance signal-to-noise ratio when identifying and characterizing event-related potentials (ERPs) or event-related magnetic fields (ERFs). These methods involve repeating the stimulus a given number of times. The recordings are then segmented into epochs, relative to the onset of each stimulus. The simplest and most commonly used procedure consists in averaging all these epochs into a single waveform. The basic assumption underlying this averaging procedure is that the stimulus-evoked activity is stationary and therefore unaffected by the averaging because its latency and morphology are invariant across all the repeated epochs. In contrast, ongoing brain activity, behaving as noise unrelated to the event, is largely cancelled out by the averaging.

The most commonly used procedure to isolate event-related brain potentials (ERPs) or event-related magnetic fields (ERFs) from background EEG or MEG is to repeat the stimulus a given number of times, to segment the continuous recordings into epochs relative to the onset of each stimulus, and to average all of these epochs into a single average waveform. The resulting waveform expresses the average signal as a function of time relative to the onset of the stimulus. Within these waveforms, reproducible changes in the signal can be assumed to reflect the synchronized activation of a population of neurons. For example, following transcutaneous electrical activation of the median nerve at the level of the wrist, the average ERP waveform includes an early negative deflection, referred to as the N20 wave (Figure 2.1, left graphs). This wave peaks approximately 20 milliseconds (ms) after the onset of the stimulus, is maximal over the central region contralateral to the stimulated hand, and reflects synchronized activation of neurons in the hand representation of S1. (Refer to Figure 2.1 in Colour Plate Section)

Hence, to reliably record ERPs or ERFs related to the perception of transient exteroceptive pain requires a method to generate nociceptive input that is sufficiently synchronous to elicit time-locked and phasic brain responses. It is for this reason that Carmon et al. introduced infrared lasers as a method to elicit ERPs related to the thermal activation of nociceptors (Carmon et al., 1976). The very steep heating ramp produced by the laser is able to bring populations of nociceptors to temperatures exceeding their thermal activation thresholds within a few milliseconds, thus generating a highly synchronous and time-locked nociceptive afferent volley.[4]

ERPS AND ERFS ELICITED BY THE CO-ACTIVATION
OF A-DELTA AND C-FIBRE NOCICEPTORS

ERPs elicited by a transient nociceptive stimulus applied against the skin predominantly consist of a large negative-positive potential, maximal at the scalp vertex, and referred to as the N2-P2 complex (Bromm & Treede, 1984; Garcia-Larrea et al., 2003) (Figure 2.2A).

The N2-P2 complex is often preceded by an earlier negative deflection, referred to as the N1 wave (Hu, Mouraux, Hu, & Iannetti, 2010; Treede, Kief, Holzer, & Bromm, 1988; Treede, Meier, Kunze, & Bromm, 1988; Valentini et al., 2012). Unlike the N2-P2, the scalp topography of the N1 wave is dependent on the location of the stimulus. When stimulating the upper limb or face, the N1 wave appears maximal over central and temporal regions contralateral to the stimulated side. When stimulating the lower limb or trunk, its scalp topography becomes more medial (Valentini et al., 2012; Xu et al., 1995). This somatotopy indicates that the N1 wave reflects activity originating at least in part from S1 (Figure 2.2B).

Because of its large amplitude, the N2-P2 complex is often visible in single trials and can be characterized reliably using only a few repeated stimuli. Source analysis studies have suggested that the N2-P2 complex reflects a combination of activity originating from the left and right insula and S2, as well as the ACC (Garcia-Larrea et al., 2003). (Refer to Figure 2.2 in Colour Plate Section)

The latencies of the N1, N2, and P2 waves of nociceptive ERPs are largely determined by the peripheral conduction distance. If the stimuli are applied to the face, the hand, or the foot, the N2 wave will peak at approximately 150–200, 200–250, and 250–300 ms respectively, while the P2 wave will peak at approximately 250–300, 350–400, and 400–450 ms. Such latencies are compatible with the conduction velocity of thinly myelinated A-delta fibres. They are, however, incompatible with the slower conduction velocities of unmyelinated C fibres.

The fact that ERPs elicited by stimuli selectively activating nociceptors can be used to assess specifically the integrity of spinothalamic pathways is illustrated in Figure 2.1 (adapted from Iannetti et al., 2013). This patient presented with thermal and pinprick hypoesthesia of the left hemibody following the surgical removal of a spinal neurinoma at level C1-C2. The MRI performed two weeks after surgery shows a clear right anterolateral location. Transcutaneous electrical nerve stimulation of the left and right median nerves elicited normal and symmetrical early-latency somatosensory-evoked potentials, indicating that lemniscal pathways were preserved. In contrast, infrared laser stimulation and mechanical pinprick stimulation elicited normal nociceptive ERPs following stimulation of the right hand but elicited abnormal ERPs following stimulation of the left hand. These results are compatible with impaired transmission of mechanical and thermal nociceptive input within the right spinothalamic tract.

The comparison of nociceptive ERPs, recorded using EEG, to nociceptive ERFs, recorded using MEG, reveals several notable differences. ERFs elicited by a transient nociceptive stimulus mainly consist of an early peak of activity whose latency closely resembles that of the early N1 wave of nociceptive ERPs (Kakigi et al., 1995). In contrast, little or no activity is observed at the latencies corresponding to the later N2-P2 complex. These differences are probably related to the fact that MEG is largely insensitive to deep sources of activity (e.g., activity originating from opercular-insular cortices and the cingulate), while it could capture superficial sources more accurately and more reliably (e.g., activity originating from S1). In addition, it is often stated that EEG signals mainly reflect sources of electrocortical activity that are radial relative to the scalp surface, whereas MEG signals mainly reflect sources of electrocortical activity that are tangential relative to the scalp surface (Hämäläinen, Hari, Ilmoniemi, Knuutila, & Lounasmaa, 1993).

ERPS AND ERFS ELICITED BY THE SELECTIVE ACTIVATION OF C FIBRE NOCICEPTORS

A number of studies have examined the ERPs and ERFs elicited by the selective thermal activation of C fibre nociceptors, using various methods to avoid the concomitant activation of A-delta nociceptors, or to block the transmission of A-delta fibre input at peripheral level (Plaghki & Mouraux, 2002). Regardless of the method used, all of these studies have confirmed that when C fibre nociceptive input is not preceded by A-delta fibre nociceptive input, the C fibre afferent volley elicits an ultra-late ERP appearing as a negative-positive complex whose latency (e.g., 750–1150 ms after stimulation of the hand) is compatible with the conduction velocity of unmyelinated C fibres. The morphology and scalp topography of these ultra-late responses closely resemble the morphology and scalp topography of the N2-P2 complex elicited by A-delta fibres. In addition, Valeriani et al. (2002) reported that the selective activation of C fibre nociceptors also elicits an earlier negative component, whose scalp topography would be similar to that of the N1 wave preceding the A-delta fibre N2-P2 complex. Indeed, just as the N1 wave related to A-delta fibres, this ultra-late N1 was described as having a lateralized scalp topography, maximal over the temporal region contralateral to the location of the stimulus on the body.

A small number of studies have used MEG to characterize the ERFs elicited by the selective activation of C fibre nociceptors (Forss, Raij, Seppa, & Hari, 2005; Kakigi et al., 2003; Qiu et al., 2004; Tran et al., 2002). The elicited responses were hypothesized to reflect the bilateral activation of opercular regions. Furthermore, with the exception of Forss et al. (2005), all of these studies included a dipole whose location was compatible with activity originating from the contralateral S1. Therefore, the sources contributing to C fibre ERFs appear to be very similar to the sources contributing to A-delta fibre ERFs.

Several studies have recorded local field potentials (LFPs) elicited by transient nociceptive stimuli within different areas of the brain of awake humans, using surgically implanted intracranial electrodes or subdural electrode grids (Peyron et al., 2002). These studies have demonstrated that brief thermal stimuli above the thermal activation threshold of A-delta and C fibres elicit responses in the left and right suprasylvian opercular region (Frot & Mauguiere, 1999, 2003; Frot, Rambaud, Guenot, & Mauguiere, 1999). The latency of the response coincides with the latency of the N1 and N2 waves of nociceptive ERPs. Interestingly, researchers observed a delay of approximately 15 ms between the responses elicited in the ipsilateral and contralateral hemispheres. Furthermore, the studies showed that thermal stimuli probably elicit two temporally distinct responses within the suprasylvian region: an early response originating from the parietal operculum, followed by a later response originating from the insula.

Attempts have also been made to record nociceptive LFPs from S1. Using subdural grids, Kanda et al. (2000) found that laser stimuli elicit a response in the contralateral S1. However, contrary to the responses elicited by non-nociceptive tactile stimuli, there was no polarity reversal when crossing the central sulcus, suggesting that the S1 response to nociceptive stimuli does not originate from the posterior bank of the central sulcus (Brodmann area 3b) and that, instead, it may originate from the depth of the central sulcus or the post-central gyrus (Brodmann area 3a or 1). Similar observations were also reported by Baumgartner et al. (2011) and Frot et al. (2012).

Several studies have attempted to record nociceptive LFPs in other regions of the awake human brain. In a recent study, Liu et al. (2010) showed that laser stimuli elicit consistent bilateral responses in the amygdala. Using subdural grids, Lenz et al. (1998) obtained reproducible biphasic responses in the mid portion of the anterior cingulate in three epileptic patients when stimulating the face at a location compatible with Brodmann area 24. However, they were unable to explain why they failed to elicit similar responses when stimulating the upper limb. Frot et al. (2008) reported that laser stimulation of the upper limb elicits consistent responses in the posterior midcingulate cortex.

Functional neuroimaging

As compared to scalp electroencephalography and the recording of scalp ERPs, functional neuroimaging offers the general advantages of higher spatial resolution and less uncertainty concerning which brain structures generate the elicited brain responses (Box 2). However, these non-invasive approaches also have disadvantages, including their low temporal resolution and the fact that they constitute an indirect measure of neural activity, related to neurovascular coupling (Arthurs & Boniface, 2002; DiNuzzo, 2014).

Box 2: Brain activity sampled using PET and fMRI

PET is a technique that relies on a measure of the concentration of a short-lived radioactive tracer isotope within a given body volume. The radioactive isotope is usually injected into the bloodstream. The physical variable that is measured by the PET camera is the distribution of radioactivity within the scanned volume. This distribution will depend on the physiological processes that are associated with the molecule carrying the positron-emitting isotope. A common use of PET is to tag water molecules and thereby obtain information concerning stimulus-induced changes in regional cerebral blood flow (rCBF). These stimulus-induced changes in rCBF are due to the phenomenon of neurovascular coupling, whose mechanism involves a complex interaction between the population of neurons activated by the stimulus and the surrounding glial and vascular cells, leading to a transient and spatially-circumscribed increase of rCBF. Typically, in so-called "activation" studies, brain areas involved in a given neural process are identified by performing a statistical comparison of the rCBF values obtained in two or more experimental conditions (e.g., the rCBF measured in the absence or presence of the stimulus, or the rCBF measured in the presence of a painful versus non-painful stimulus).

The majority of fMRI studies aiming at characterizing the brain responses related to the perception of pain rely on assessing stimulus-related changes in BOLD signal. The BOLD signal is dependent on the ratio between oxygenated and deoxygenated hemoglobin. The inflow of oxyhemoglobin due to the increase in rCBF induced by neurovascular coupling largely overcompensates the increase in oxygen extraction due to metabolic demands. The bulk of the effect of neural activation is thus a regional increase of the oxyhemoglobin/deoxyhemoglobin ratio.

In the field of pain, the majority of PET and fMRI studies have focused on comparing the brain responses (i.e., the changes in rCBF) triggered by nociceptive versus non-nociceptive stimuli and/or stimuli perceived as painful versus not painful. To generate the stimuli, most studies have relied on contact thermodes. Some studies have relied on a relatively long-lasting thermal stimulus (e.g., 30 seconds), whereas other studies have relied on brief transient thermal stimuli applied repetitively. A fewer number of studies have relied on laser stimulation. These different studies have shown that nociceptive stimuli, or stimuli perceived as painful, elicit a significant increase of rCBF in a large number of brain regions, including the insula, S1, S2, the ACC, the thalamus, the dorsolateral prefrontal cortex, the midbrain, and the cerebellum (Bushnell & Apkarian, 2006; Talbot et al., 1991) (Figure 2.3, upper panel). (Refer to Figure 2.3 in Colour Plate Section)

Where is the primary nociceptive cortex?

In most sensory modalities, investigators have been able to clearly delineate a cortical area devoted specifically to receiving and processing the primary thalamocortical projections belonging to that particular sensory modality. For example, auditory input projects onto the primary auditory cortex, visual input onto the primary visual cortex, and somatosensory input onto the primary somatosensory cortex. In contrast, nociceptive input does not appear to project onto a cortical area devoted exclusively to receiving and processing nociceptive input (i.e., a primary nociceptive cortex) (Andersson & Rydenhag, 1985; Iannetti & Mouraux, 2010). Indeed, regardless of the method used to measure brain activity, no cortical area specifically involved in the processing of ascending nociceptive input has ever been clearly isolated. Instead, nociceptive-specific neurons (i.e., neurons responding exclusively to the activation of nociceptors) appear to be disseminated in cortical structures that are also involved in processing non-nociceptive sensory input and/or that are also involved in other higher-order brain functions. The fact that the cortical representation of nociception does not appear to involve neurons spatially organized in a nociceptive-specific cortical area puts into question the commonly accepted notion that nociception constitutes a distinct sensory system.

Involvement of S1 in the perception of transient exteroceptive pain

The involvement of S1 in the processing of nociceptive input and the perception of pain is controversial (Apkarian et al., 2005; Bushnell et al., 1999; Liang, Mouraux, & Iannetti, 2011; Mountcastle, 2005; Ploner, Schmitz, Freund, & Schnitzler, 1999). Some authors have suggested that S1 is the primary target for ascending nociceptive input of the spinothalamic pathway. Others have suggested that S1 plays a trivial role in pain perception. Although extensive lesions of S1 have been shown to induce a transient deficit in pain perception, patients with long-standing lesions show little or no deficits (Head & Holmes, 1911). Furthermore, direct electrical stimulation of S1 does not appear to elicit pain. However, some authors have reported that focal epileptic crises involving S1 can, in some rare cases, generate pain-related experiences (Young & Blume, 1983).

Mountcastle (1957) showed that neurons in S1 are organized in "cortical columns" containing neurons having similar receptive fields and response properties, which he proposed constituted an "elementary unit of organization". Neurons responding to nociceptive stimuli are not organized in distinct columns. Instead, somatosensory cortical columns can contain neurons driven by non-nociceptive input as well as neurons driven by nociceptive input (Kenshalo, Iwata, Sholas, & Thomas, 2000).

Most importantly, the most common finding across studies is that S1 neurons responding specifically to nociceptive stimuli are very sparse.[5] Furthermore, the responses of the few nociceptive-specific neurons that have been identified in S1 are often too slow to be considered as the neuronal activity from which pain emerges (Tommerdahl, Delemos, Vierck, Favorov, & Whitsel, 1996; Whitsel, Favorov, Li, Quibrera, & Tommerdahl, 2009). In conditions of central sensitization these neurons may also respond to low-intensity stimuli, which suggests that they are not strictly specific for nociception. Wall (1995) concluded that, "it remains an act of faith to continue searching the brain and spinal cord for some still undiscovered nest of cells whose activity reliably triggers pain." In fact, one may wonder whether the identification of nociceptive-specific neurons does not constitute an epiphenomenon resulting simply from the variable and varying activation thresholds of neurons.

Whether or not S1 plays an important role in the processing of nociceptive input thus remains an open question. In particular, there is still no unequivocal evidence demonstrating an obligatory involvement of S1 in extracting the sensory-discriminative dimension of pain perception (i.e., a role in evaluating the intensity, localization, and duration of a nociceptive stimulus) – although this has often been postulated by researchers.

Functional neuroimaging studies and electrophysiological studies in humans have shown that transient exteroceptive nociceptive stimuli can elicit activity in the contralateral S1 (Bingel et al., 2004; Bushnell et al., 1999; Hu, Valentini, Zhang, Liang, & Iannetti, 2014; Talbot et al., 1991; Valentini et al., 2012). However, this is not systematically observed across studies, suggesting that the S1 response to nociceptive stimulation may be strongly dependent on contextual factors. One possibility is that the bulk of the responses in S1 following nociceptive stimulation is not strictly related to processing ascending nociceptive input and, instead, relates to the fact that a nociceptive stimulus applied at a given location is likely to attract attention towards that location. In other words, changes in S1 activity following nociceptive stimulation might mainly reflect the fact that the nociceptive stimulus triggers a top-down attentional modulation of S1 (Jones, Friston, & Frackowiak, 1992).

It is generally accepted that non-nociceptive somatosensory input, such as vibrotactile input, is predominantly processed in a serial fashion from the thalamus to S1, and from S1 to other brain regions such as S2 (Allison et al., 1989a; Allison, McCarthy, Wood, Williamson, & Spencer, 1989b; Mountcastle, 2005). Several studies have suggested that, in contrast to this serial organization, nociceptive input projects in parallel from the thalamus to S1, S2, and other brain regions such as the insula and the ACC (Kanda et al., 2000; Ploner et al., 1999). However, empirical evidence supporting this notion is still lacking (Liang et al., 2011).

Involvement of the operculo-insular cortex in the perception of transient exteroceptive pain

The most consistent finding across human brain imaging studies is that nociceptive stimuli elicit bilateral activation of the operculo-insular cortex, including S2, the posterior insula, and the anterior insula (Bushnell & Apkarian, 2006; Garcia-Larrea et al., 2003; Ingvar, 1999; Peyron et al., 2000; Porro, 2003; Tracey & Mantyh, 2007; Treede et al., 1999). Furthermore, as detailed previously, robust activation within these regions has also been confirmed using intracerebral recordings performed in humans for the diagnostic workup of focal intractable epilepsy. Further supporting a strong involvement of these areas in the processing of nociceptive input is the evidence that focal epileptic activity involving these brain structures, as well as direct electrical stimulation of these brain structures (in particular, the posterior insula) can, in some patients, generate pain-related experiences (Charlesworth, Soryal, Smith, & Sisodiya, 2009; Isnard, Guenot, Sindou, & Mauguiere, 2004; Ostrowsky et al., 2002; Young & Blume, 1983). In addition, lesions of the insula have been reported to impair the ability to perceive pain (Greenspan, Lee, & Lenz, 1999; Greenspan & Winfield, 1992). Taken together, these observations suggest a major role for the operculo-insular cortex in pain perception, leading some authors to suggest that the posterior insula and surrounding opercular cortex could constitute some form of "primary nociceptive cortex" (Craig, Chen, Bandy, & Reiman, 2000; Garcia-Larrea, 2012; Garcia-Larrea & Peyron, 2013).

However, there are also strong counterarguments to this hypothesis.

First, the insula is implicated in the processing of a wide range of sensory inputs and contributes to a large number of cognitive, affective, interoceptive, and homeostatic functions, independent of sensory modality (zu Eulenburg, Baumgartner, Treede, & Dieterich, 2013). This is not surprising, given the wide spectrum of anatomical connections and the heterogeneous cytoarchitecture of the insula (Cauda & Vercelli, 2013). Therefore, the robust responses triggered by nociceptive stimuli in the insula could, at least in part, be unspecific for nociception and unrelated to the actual perception of pain. For example, the insula is thought to play an important role in the detection of salience (i.e., the property of a stimulus that causes it to stand out relative to neighboring stimuli) (Downar, Crawley, Mikulis, & Davis, 2000; Downar, Crawley, Mikulis, & Davis, 2002) and possibly constitutes a hub connecting sensory areas to other networks involved in the processing and integration of external and internal information. Such connections would allow the generation of a coherent representation of different salient conditions including, but not limited to, pain-related conditions (Liang, Mouraux, & Iannetti, 2013b).

Second, direct electrical stimulation of the insula does not always elicit pain. Ostrowsky et al. (2002) found that pain-related sensations were elicited in only 17 out of 93 insular stimulation sites, and in only 14 patients out of 43. Furthermore, in the majority of cases, the stimuli also elicited non-painful somesthetic sensations, leading the authors to conclude that, "painful and non-painful somesthetic representations in the human insula overlap."

Third, although pain is a recognized manifestation of epileptic seizures, its occurrence is actually uncommon (less than 3% in a series of 858 epileptic patients) (Young & Blume, 1983). Furthermore, pain is virtually never the sole manifestation of a seizure. Instead, ictal pain is most often associated with the perception of non-painful paraesthesias, thermal sensations, or a disturbance of somatognosia.

Finally, although there are several case reports suggesting that lesions of the insula can alter pain perception, there are also case reports showing the opposite (Baier et al., 2014; Feinstein et al., 2015). For example, Feinstein et al. (2015) recently reported the case of a patient with extensive bilateral damage of the operculo-insular region who had no marked deficit in the ability to perceive pain.

The pain matrix as a biomarker for pain perception?

Probably because researchers have failed to identify a spatially-segregated cortical area devoted exclusively to processing nociceptive input, several authors have proposed that the perception of pain emerges from the joint activation of a *network* of brain structures. This network would encompass all structures shown to be consistently activated following nociceptive stimulation, particularly somatosensory areas (S1, S2), the insula, and the ACC (Garcia-Larrea & Peyron, 2013; Tracey & Mantyh, 2007).

It has been repeatedly demonstrated that, within this "pain matrix," the magnitude of the brain responses elicited by a transient exteroceptive nociceptive can correlate robustly with the intensity of perceived pain (Coghill et al., 1999; Derbyshire et al., 1997; Iannetti, Zambreanu, Cruccu, & Tracey, 2005; Tolle et al., 1999). These observations have led some authors to conclude that these brain responses support the encoding of pain intensity (Porro, 2003; Rainville, 2002). In addition, this has led some authors to propose that the magnitude of the brain responses in the pain matrix could be used as a *biomarker for pain* (Schweinhardt et al., 2006; Segerdahl, Mezue, Okell, Farrar, & Tracey, 2015).

Using various experimental manipulations, studies have also shown that it is possible to differentially modulate the magnitude of pain-evoked responses in different subregions of the pain matrix. This finding has been interpreted as evidence that different subregions of this network may process different aspects of the pain experience (Ingvar, 1999). For example, hypnotic suggestion of increased intensity of perceived pain has been shown to selectively increase the response magnitude in somatosensory areas, whereas hypnotic suggestion of increased pain unpleasantness may selectively increase the response magnitude in the ACC (Hofbauer, Rainville, Duncan, & Bushnell, 2001; Rainville, Duncan, Price, Carrier, & Bushnell, 1997).

When interpreting the functional significance of the brain responses evoked by nociceptive stimuli, initial reports have been extremely cautious (Carmon et al., 1976; Chapman, Chen, Colpitts, & Martin, 1981; Stowell, 1984). For example, in his seminal paper introducing laser-evoked brain potentials as a technique to explore nociception in humans, Carmon et al. (1976) concluded that, "it is possible that only the arousing and alerting effect of pain is responsible for the electroencephalographic phenomenon observed."

As an increasing number of studies showed that nociceptive stimuli, or stimuli perceived as painful, elicit consistent responses within the pain matrix and that the magnitude of these responses correlates with the perception of pain, several investigators began to consider that it is reasonable to assume that the elicited brain responses are specific for pain. This conclusion is based on common reasoning in functional neuroimaging referred to as *reverse inference* (Poldrack, 2006; Yarkoni, Poldrack, Nichols, Van Essen, & Wager, 2011). The finding that a given mental state (e.g., the perception of pain) is commonly associated with the activation of a given brain structure (e.g., the pain matrix) leads to the conclusion that this mental state emerges from the activation of that structure. However, the validity of this reasoning is dependent on the exclusivity of the relationship between the mental state and the activated brain structure. If the pain matrix is also activated by a variety of mental states other than pain, then it is likely that the pain matrix reflects cognitive processes that are unrelated to the actual experience of pain (Iannetti, Salomons, Moayedi, Mouraux, & Davis, 2013).

There are, in fact, a number of arguments indicating that the pain matrix does not reflect cortical activity specifically involved in the perception of pain.

First, although a common observation is that the magnitude of the responses in the pain matrix correlates with the intensity of pain perception, an increasing number of studies have shown that, in specific experimental conditions, the pain matrix response can be entirely dissociated from pain perception (Chapman et al., 1981; Clark, Brown, Jones, & El-Deredy, 2008; Dillmann, Miltner, & Weiss, 2000; Iannetti, Hughes, Lee, & Mouraux, 2008; Lee, Mouraux, & Iannetti, 2009; Mouraux, Guerit, & Plaghki, 2004; Mouraux & Plaghki, 2007). For example, Iannetti et al. (2008) delivered trains of three identical nociceptive stimuli with a constant one-second interstimulus interval, using four different stimulation intensities. As expected, the magnitude of the brain response elicited by the first stimulus correlated strongly with the energy of the eliciting stimulus and the intensity of perceived pain. However, for the responses elicited by the second and third stimuli, this relationship was markedly disrupted: stimulus repetition significantly decreased the magnitude of the elicited brain responses, although it did not affect pain perception. Similarly, Clark et al. (2008) presented nociceptive stimuli cued by a preceding visual signal. They observed that the duration of the delay separating the onset of the cue and the onset of the nociceptive stimulus affected differently the magnitude of the brain response elicited by the nociceptive stimulus and the intensity of pain perception. Longer delays led to increased ratings of pain perception. In contrast, the magnitude of the elicited brain responses depended on whether the delay was predictable: the brain responses were increased when the delay was unpredictable, regardless of the duration of the delay.

Additional evidence that activation of the pain matrix can be dissociated from pain perception is provided by studies showing that nociceptive stimuli can generate a perception of pain without eliciting any measurable brain response in the pain matrix. For example, when brief thermal stimuli are applied to the skin, such as to co-activate fast-conducting myelinated A-delta nociceptors and slow-conducting unmyelinated C nociceptors, this leads to the perception of two temporally-distinct sensations referred to as "first pain" and "second pain." However, the EEG responses to such a stimulus only show activity related to the activation of A-delta nociceptors (see Section 2.2.1). Conversely, if the concomitant activation of A-delta nociceptors is avoided, the selective activation of C fibres elicits both an isolated perception of second pain and a measurable brain response within the pain matrix.

In a series of two studies using EEG and fMRI (Figures 2.2 and 2.3), the brain responses elicited by nociceptive stimuli inducing a perception of pain were compared to the brain responses elicited by non-nociceptive somatosensory, auditory, and visual stimuli (Mouraux, Diukova, Lee, Wise, & Iannetti, 2011a; Mouraux, Gille, Dorban, & Peeters, 2002; Mouraux & Iannetti, 2009). It is important to note that all stimuli were presented in a random sequence, using a large and unpredictable interstimulus interval, in order to maximize their salience. In the first study (Figure 2.2), a blind source separation technique was used to decompose the EEG responses elicited by the different types of stimuli into a set of physiologically independent components. The analysis showed that the bulk of nociceptive ERPs could be explained by multimodal neural activity also contributing to the ERPs elicited by non-nociceptive somatosensory, auditory, and visual stimuli (Figure 2.2A). Source analysis of these components showed that they could originate from bilateral operculo-insular regions as well as from the ACC (Figure 2.2C). In addition to this multimodal activity, somatosensory-specific activity was found to contribute to the early-latency components of both nociceptive and non-nociceptive somatosensory ERPs. Strikingly, no nociceptive-specific activity could be identified, suggesting that although nociceptive ERPs are related specifically to the activation of peripheral nociceptors, they do not reflect cortical activity that is specific for nociception.

In the second study using fMRI (Figure 2.3), the investigators examined the BOLD activity elicited by the same stimuli and reached the same conclusion: nociceptive, somatosensory, auditory, and visual stimuli elicited spatially indistinguishable responses in the cingulate, the insula, and the largest part of S2. Furthermore, a matching pattern of activation was also observed for nociceptive and non-nociceptive somatosensory stimuli in S1 and in a small subregion of S2. Strikingly, nociceptive stimuli did not appear to elicit any specific response.

Most interestingly, the magnitude of both the multimodal component of nociceptive ERPs (Figure 2.2D) and the magnitude of multimodal BOLD responses (Figure 2.3, lower panel) was significantly correlated with subjective ratings of stimulus salience, independent of the modality of the eliciting stimuli.

Further studies are needed to understand the functional significance of these brain responses. The fact that stimulus salience appears to be one of the main determinants of these responses could suggest that they reflect cortical activity involved in the detection of salient events or in triggering responses related to the occurrence of events such as an involuntary reorientation of attention. However, at least some of these brain responses could also be related, for example, to arousal reactions, autonomic activation, or affective responses.

Nevertheless, these different results showing that pain can be perceived without activating the "pain matrix," and that the pain matrix can be activated by stimuli that do not elicit a perception of pain, indicate that these brain responses cannot be used as an "objective" biomarker for pain.

Cortical representation of tonic pain

The large body of experimental evidence showing that the cortical responses elicited by transient nociceptive stimuli largely reflect the detection and reaction to potentially dangerous environmental changes implies that such responses are not necessarily adequate to explore the neural activity underlying the actual emergence of pain. As discussed in Section 6, below, the use of novel approaches to analysis might help tease out more pain-specific brain responses. Most importantly, experimental designs involving long-lasting nociceptive stimulation that result in tonic pain sensations may constitute a promising strategy to enhance the likelihood of extracting neural activities that are more specifically related to the actual perception of pain and, possibly, that are more closely related to the pathophysiology of clinical pain conditions.

Several approaches have been developed to assess the changes in brain activity related to the experience of tonic pain.

Using EEG, studies that have attempted to characterize the changes in spontaneous EEG oscillatory activity have yielded inconsistent findings (Backonja et al., 1991; Dowman, Rissacher, & Schuckers, 2008; Huber, Bartling, Pachur, Woikowsky-Biedau, & Lautenbacher, 2006; Le Pera et al., 2000). Some studies have reported suppression of alpha-band oscillations (8–12 Hz) over frontal-central, temporal, or parietal-occipital regions. Contradicting these findings, other studies have shown increased alpha-band oscillations over frontal or parietal-occipital regions. In addition, several recent studies have shown enhanced gamma-band oscillations (GBO; >40 Hz) during the experience of tonic pain (Schulz et al., 2015). The functional significance of these changes remains largely unknown. In a recent study, Peng et al. (2014) assessed how the focus of attention affects the changes in EEG spectrum induced by tonic painful stimuli. They found that the strength of the decrease in alpha-band power induced by tonic pain was strongly dependent on the focus of attention. In contrast, the strength of the increase in gamma-band power appeared to be largely independent of attention. This dissociation suggests that alpha-band suppression and gamma-band enhancement reflect distinct processes, differentially dependent on top-down factors such as attentional state.

Also using EEG, researchers have recently attempted to characterize the cortical representation of tonic pain using an original approach based on the recording of "steady-state evoked potentials" (SS-EPs) (Colon, Legrain, & Mouraux, 2012, 2014; Mouraux et al., 2011b). Unlike conventional ERPs that reflect a phasic cortical response triggered by the occurrence of a brief stimulus, SS-EPs reflect a sustained cortical response induced by the long-lasting periodic repetition of a sensory stimulus. This cortical response is thought to result from an entrainment of neuronal populations responding to the periodically modulated feature of the stimulus (Regan, 1989). As compared to ERPs, as well as to other non-invasive approaches to record brain activity in humans such as fMRI, investigating brain function using SS-EPs offers several advantages. In other sensory modalities, it was shown that SS-EPs: (1) exhibit a particularly high signal-to-noise ratio; and (2) reflect neural activity originating mainly from modality-specific sensory cortices. Furthermore, (3) SS-EPs are probably less contaminated by stimulus-evoked cognitive processes related to arousal and attentional capture than are other non-invasive approaches.

For these reasons, Mouraux et al. (2010) developed a means to record SS-EPs related to the rapid periodic thermal activation of cutaneous nociceptors in humans. The elicited responses were maximal at the scalp vertex and symmetrically distributed over both hemispheres, suggesting a radial source originating from midline brain structures such as the ACC. This midline scalp topography contrasted strongly with the lateralized scalp topography of the SS-EPs obtained by innocuous vibrotactile stimulation, which displayed a clear maximum over the parietal region contralateral to the stimulated side, suggesting a tangential source originating from the contralateral S1. Because the spatial distribution of noxious somatosensory SS-EPs was markedly different from the spatial distribution of innocuous somatosensory SS-EPs, it was hypothesized that nociceptive SS-EPs reflect the activity of a cortical network preferentially involved in processing input conveyed by nociceptors, spatially distinct from the somatotopically organized cortical network involved in processing innocuous vibrotactile input. Future studies are clearly needed to better understand the functional significance of these brain responses.

Finally, several studies have attempted to characterize the brain responses to tonic pain using fMRI. These studies also found that tonic and phasic pain lead to differential activation patterns. For example, Ringler et al. (2003) found that phasic mechanical pain elicits strong responses in S1 and S2. In contrast, tonic pressure pain elicited little activity in somatosensory areas but induced strong activation of the ACC and frontal areas. Recently, using arterial spin-labeling, Segerdahl et al. (2015) found that the intensity of sustained pain generated by capsaicin and heat correlated specifically with the rCBF within the dorsal posterior portion of the insula.

Cortical representation of visceral pain

Most studies have focused on brain responses to exteroceptive nociceptive stimuli delivered to the skin. Less is known about the cortical processing of visceral nociceptive information, mostly because generating controlled nociceptive visceral stimulation is technically challenging. Studies have yielded contrasting results, showing overlap but also differentiation between the cortical representations of somatic and visceral pain (Dunckley et al., 2005; Mayer, Gupta, Kilpatrick, & Hong, 2015).

Cortical representation of chronic pathological pain

In an fMRI study performed with patients with chronic spontaneous back pain, Baliki et al. (2006) identified brain regions in which the BOLD signal could be predicted by the spontaneous fluctuations of pain. The brain activity related to spontaneous pain was restricted to the medial prefrontal cortex and did not show any overlap with the brain activity elicited by brief experimental thermal pain. Interestingly, spontaneous transient increases in chronic back pain did transiently elicit activity within the "pain matrix," suggesting that the pain matrix may be specifically related to the experience of acute pain, and/or that it reflects cognitive or affective processes resulting from the experience of acute pain. In other words, the finding that the pain matrix is not activated during spontaneous chronic pain could be due to the fact that it is not so much involved in pain perception. Or it could be due to the fact that the cortical representation of pain may change over time (prolonged pain experience could lead to activity-dependent changes in the cortical representation of pain). Regardless, these observations indicate that activity measured in the pain matrix cannot be considered as a surrogate for measuring pain in patients.

Other approaches to characterize the cortical representation of pain

Functional connectivity and resting state networks

There is currently a general agreement that in order to progress in our understanding of how pain is represented in the human brain we will need to be able to better characterize the functional connectivity, interdependency, and hierarchical organization of the different brain regions responding to noxious input. This will help us to appreciate how noxious information propagates within these different brain regions and how these brain regions interact with each other to generate painful percepts and pain-related behaviors (Bingel & Tracey, 2008). Furthermore, it has been suggested that changes in functional connectivity could constitute a key pathophysiological mechanism underlying certain states of chronic pain (Apkarian, Baliki, & Farmer, 2013).

Several studies have attempted to address these questions using methods such as Dynamic Causal Modeling (Liang et al., 2011) to assess functional connectivity based on fMRI data. However, interpretation of the results obtained using these techniques is undermined by the fact that the low temporal resolution of BOLD signals precludes determining whether functional connectivity between two regions reflects a direct connection or an indirect connection involving multiple intervening regions (Greicius, Supekar, Menon, & Dougherty, 2009). In addition, correlation measurements performed using BOLD signals could at least partly be influenced by fluctuations in cerebral metabolism and blood flow unrelated to the elicited neural activity (Fukunaga et al., 2008). A smaller number of studies have attempted to assess functional connectivity using EEG or MEG data (e.g., Ploner, Schoffelen, Schnitzler, & Gross, 2009). However, this also has significant drawbacks due mainly to the low spatial resolution of the recorded signals.

In addition to measuring the functional connectivity between brain regions responding to a sensory stimulus, or brain regions activated during the performance of a given task, it is also possible to measure functional connectivity during "rest" (Biswal, Yetkin, Haughton, & Hyde, 1995). Without external stimulation, the human brain spontaneously produces low-frequency fluctuations of activity. These spontaneous fluctuations show a high degree of correlation across separated brain regions, indicating that they may reflect networks of functionally-connected brain regions, such as the "default mode network," the "salience network," and the "sensorimotor network" (Cordes et al., 2000; Hampson, Peterson, Skudlarski, Gatenby, & Gore, 2002; Seeley et al., 2007). However, interpreting differences across conditions or between groups of subjects is not straightforward (Cole, Smith, & Beckmann, 2010). Observed differences could be related to changes in the connectivity of the networks but could also be related to instructed or self-initiated changes in mental state. For example, being instructed to "rest" and refrain from moving in an fMRI scanner may lead to a very different mental state in patients experiencing pain as compared to healthy controls. Furthermore, differences in resting-state functional connectivity are difficult to disentangle from fluctuations in BOLD signals due to physiological (respiratory, cardiac, vasomotor) and motion confounds.

Despite these limitations, several studies have identified links between changes in these resting-state networks and the experience of pain. For example, in a recent longitudinal study of patients presenting with subacute back pain, Baliki et al. (2012) found that functional connectivity between the nucleus accumbens and the medial prefrontal cortex was higher in patients who would develop persistent back pain as compared to patients who would recover from their back pain. These observations, as well as those of other studies, indicate that differences or changes in functional connectivity could help us to identify different pain states in humans.

Pain-related changes in neuro-oscillatory activity

In addition to ERPs, transient nociceptive stimuli also induce changes in the magnitude of ongoing EEG oscillations (Mouraux et al., 2003; Ohara, Crone, Weiss, Treede, & Lenz, 2004; Ploner, Gross, Timmermann, Pollok, & Schnitzler, 2006; Zhang, Hu, Hung, Mouraux, & Iannetti, 2012). These changes consist of a short-lasting and early-latency enhancement of signal power at frequencies around 10 Hz, followed by a long-lasting reduction of signal power within the same frequency band. In addition, several studies have shown that nociceptive stimulation induces a transient and early-latency enhancement of GBO (40–100 Hz) (Gross, Schnitzler, Timmermann, & Ploner, 2007; Zhang et al., 2012). In contrast to nociceptive ERPs, the magnitude of GBOs appears to correlate with the intensity of pain perception regardless of factors, such as stimulus repetition, modulating stimulus salience. This suggests that stimulus-induced GBOs could reflect cortical activity more directly related to the perception of pain (Zhang et al., 2012). When stimulating the hand, GBOs appear to be maximal over the central region contralateral to the stimulated hand, suggesting that these responses could originate from S1 (or from the primary motor cortex) (Schulz et al., 2015; Zhang et al., 2012). Further data is clearly required to determine whether these responses can be assessed reliably at single-subject level, to confirm their cortical origin, and to further characterize the relationship between these responses and perception – for example, in the context of sustained pain.

Multivariate analyses and cerebral signatures for pain

The fact that experiencing pain is associated with complex and distributed patterns of brain activity has led several researchers to examine whether multivariate approaches, such as multivariate pattern analysis (MVPA), could identify spatial patterns of brain activity specifically related to the experience of pain (Liang, Mouraux, Hu, & Iannetti, 2013a; Wager et al., 2013). Such data-driven "mind reading" approaches have become very popular over the past years because they could lead to a method for studying brain function using a more holistic approach.

MVPA is a machine-learning technique that uses a pattern classifier to identify the *representational content* of the fMRI responses elicited, for example, by different types of sensory stimuli (Kriegeskorte, Goebel, & Bandettini, 2006; Mur, Bandettini, & Kriegeskorte, 2009). Whereas conventional univariate approaches attempt to link a given experimental variable to the activity measured within a single voxel or a single cluster of voxels, multivariate approaches attempt to link the experimental variable to patterns of activity across many voxels. Considering the responses elicited by a sensory stimulus, MVPA can be used to test whether the stimulus elicits a specific spatial pattern of activity across the multiple voxels of a given brain region. It is generally considered that MVPA is more sensitive than conventional univariate analysis in disclosing fine within-region spatial differences in brain activity across experimental conditions. Specifically, MVPA may be able to detect changes in the spatial distribution of BOLD signals even when regional-average activity does not differ across the conditions. For these reasons, some authors have proposed that MVPA can be used to disclose a *cerebral signature* for pain – that is, a spatial pattern of brain activity that would be specific to the experience of pain (Wager et al., 2013).

MVPA takes the form of solving a classification problem – for example, guessing whether a given fMRI response is related to the perception of pain or touch. For this purpose, the fMRI data is divided into a *training* dataset and a *test* dataset. The training dataset is used to train the classifier that learns the spatial pattern of the responses elicited in each experimental condition. The trained classifier is then applied to the test dataset to assess its ability to predict the stimulus eliciting the response. If the predictions made by the classifier are above chance level, this implies that the different experimental conditions elicit distinct spatial patterns of fMRI activity.

It is important to distinguish *within-subject* MVPA from *between-subject* MVPA, as they address fundamentally different questions. In within-subject MVPA, the classifier is trained on the fMRI data of a single subject and tested on remaining fMRI data of that same subject. Therefore, within-subject MVPA examines whether the different experimental conditions elicit distinct spatial patterns of brain activity at the single-subject level, regardless of whether these spatial patterns are consistent across subjects. In between-subject MVPA, the classifier is trained on the fMRI data of a group of subjects. Therefore, between-subject MVPA requires spatially-distinct patterns of brain activity that are consistent across subjects. Considering the presence of interindividual anatomical variation, as well as inevitable coregistration errors, activated areas across subjects are unlikely to be represented in exactly the same voxels. Hence, between-subject MVPA is likely to distinguish spatial patterns of brain activity if these are distinct at regional level, but not at voxel level.

Recently, several studies have shown that these machine-learning techniques can successfully predict the intensity of pain perception using both fMRI signals (Wager et al., 2013) and EEG signals (Huang et al., 2013). In these between-subject studies, nociceptive stimuli of different intensities were delivered to healthy participants and a predictor was successfully derived from the fMRI or EEG data to predict the level of perceived pain. This led the authors to conclude that these multivariate approaches could be used as an "objective measure of pain." However, this conclusion is undermined by the same weakness regarding the validity of the reverse inference (see previous section). Hence, as the results of univariate analyses show a relationship between the magnitude of the brain responses elicited by a nociceptive stimulus and the intensity of pain perception, the ability of multivariate analyses to predict the level of perceived pain could be explained by the fact that pain intensity covaries with other features of the stimulus, such as its salience. Therefore, it is unknown whether these patterns actually constitute a *signature for pain* or whether they constitute a *multimodal signature* related, for example, to stimulus salience.

Interestingly, using within-subject MVPA, which is more likely to capture fine-grained differences in the spatial patterns of BOLD responses sampled in a single subject, it was recently shown that unique signatures for pain, but also unique signatures for touch, audition, and vision, can be identified within the different brain regions constituting the so-called pain matrix (Liang et al., 2013a). Most interestingly, within-subject MVPA also showed that pain, touch, audition, and vision elicit spatially-distinct patterns of brain activity in all primary sensory cortices. For example, the spatial distribution of the fMRI signals measured in the primary visual cortex enabled researchers to distinguish between tactile and nociceptive stimuli above chance level.

Sampling brain activity to assess pain in patients with disorders of consciousness

Although there is now accumulating evidence that the bulk of the brain responses elicited by stimuli perceived as painful do not reflect activity that is specific for nociception or the perception of pain, and that the magnitude of these brain responses does not necessarily correlate with the intensity of pain perception, the ability to record such brain responses could constitute a highly useful tool for inferring whether patients who are unable to communicate may have the ability to perceive pain or whether they are actually experiencing pain at a given moment in time.

Using PET, Laureys et al. (2002) investigated the brain activity of patients in a vegetative state following the delivery of transcutaneous electrical stimuli to the median nerve using an intensity that elicited a clear perception of pain in healthy individuals. Laureys et al. (2002) observed significant activation of the midbrain, contralateral thalamus, and S1, but not of the other brain regions commonly activated by stimuli eliciting pain. This contrasted with the results obtained in healthy controls, in which the same stimuli elicited significant activity in the midbrain, contralateral thalamus, and S1, but also in S2, the insula, and the ACC. Because transcutaneous electrical stimulation does not activate nociceptors selectively, it could well be that at least part of the elicited brain activity was related to the processing of non-nociceptive somatosensory input conveyed by the medial lemniscus pathway (in particular, the isolated S1 response in patients). Nevertheless, the lack of activity in cortical structures other than S1 could indicate that, in these patients, the painful electrical stimuli did not elicit a conscious percept. Slightly different results were obtained by Kassubek et al. (2003). They also used PET to study the brain responses to a similar electrical stimulus in seven patients in a post-anoxic vegetative state and found significant activation in S1, S2, the posterior insula, and the ACC (i.e., those brain regions that have been shown to be consistently activated by pain in healthy individuals). Although there is accumulating evidence challenging the notion that activity within these brain regions is directly related to the perception of pain, the finding that noxious stimulation elicited widespread cortical activity in this group of patients does suggest residual ability to experience pain. Most importantly, the finding that painful electrical stimuli can elicit different patterns of subcortical and cortical responses in different groups of patients with disorders of consciousness suggests that functional brain imaging might be useful to identify patients more or less likely to perceive pain following nociceptive stimulation.

In a subsequent study, Boly et al. (2008) used PET to compare the brain activity elicited by painful electrical stimuli in five patients in a minimally conscious state (MCS), 15 patients in persistent vegetative state (PVS), and 15 healthy controls. In patients in MCS and in the healthy controls, the stimuli elicited a similar pattern of brain activity in regions including the thalamus, S1, S2, the insula, and the ACC. As compared to patients in MCS and the healthy controls, patients in PVS showed significantly reduced activity in S1, S2, the insula, and the ACC. Again, these results are compatible with the notion that functional brain imaging could be able to distinguish different groups of patients with disorders of consciousness who have differing abilities to experience pain.

Using fMRI, Markl et al. (2013) compared the patterns of brain activity elicited by painful electrical stimuli in 30 patients in PVS and 15 age-matched healthy controls, using an alternating block design (60 seconds of stimulation alternating with 60 seconds of rest). Activation of S1 was observed in only 3/30 PVS patients. Activation of S2 (5/30), the anterior insula (5/30), and/ or the ACC (5/30) was also reported in some patients. Importantly, significant activation of these regions was more frequently, but not systematically, observed in the healthy controls. For example, significant activation of the ACC was observed in only 6/15 healthy controls.

In a series of recent studies, de Tommaso et al. (2013; 2015) recorded ERPs elicited by transient laser stimuli selectively activating heat-sensitive nociceptors in patients in MCS, patients in PVS, and healthy age-matched controls. In all patients, including those in PVS, the nociceptive stimuli elicited a measurable ERP whose scalp topography was compatible with activity originating from the "pain matrix."

These EEG results contrast markedly with the results of functional neuroimaging studies conducted using PET and fMRI. The different results could, of course, be related to differences in the patient populations studied, or to differences in the nature of the brain activity sampled by PET, fMRI, and EEG. However, they could also be explained by the use of different methods to elicit pain. In the studies of de Tommaso et al. (2013, 2015), pain-related brain responses were obtained using an infrared laser stimulus known to selectively and reliably activate heat-sensitive nociceptive afferents. In contrast, previous PET and fMRI studies have all relied on transcutaneous electrical stimuli that may not have been of a sufficient intensity to reliably activate nociceptive afferents.

Interestingly, de Tommaso et al. (2015) found that, unlike nociceptive laser stimuli, non-nociceptive somatosensory, auditory, and visual stimuli did not elicit reproducible late-latency ERPs in most patients in MCS. They interpreted this as resulting from the fact that nociceptive input may be intrinsically more salient than non-nociceptive input.

All of these different studies have aimed at assessing the ability of patients with disorders of consciousness to perceive pain elicited by a noxious stimulus. However, they do not address the fact that these patients may experience spontaneous pain in the absence of external stimulation or that they may experience pain elicited by innocuous stimuli. The nociceptive system has an exquisite ability to sensitize following lesions of itself, leading to neuropathic pain. The function of the peripheral and central mechanisms leading to sensitization could be to compensate for a reduced ability to transmit and respond to nociceptive input. Neuropathic pain is thus characterized by the combination of chronic pain and an impaired ability to respond to external nociceptive stimuli – as demonstrated, for example, by reduced or altered brain responses to experimental nociceptive stimuli such as laser-evoked brain potentials (Figure 2.1).

Whether the brain lesions leading to disorders of consciousness could also lead to unrecognized states of neuropathic pain should thus be considered. In these patients, one would actually expect reduced brain responses to nociceptive stimulation. There is currently a large amount of research aiming at developing methods to assess spontaneous ongoing pain in humans by, for example, demonstrating activity-dependent changes in connectivity or differences in the magnitude of brain oscillations. Hopefully, these techniques will one day make it possible to assess spontaneous pain in humans, including patients with disorders of consciousness.

Notes

1 **André Mouraux** is Professor at the Faculty of Medicine of the Université catholique de Louvain, Institute of Neuroscience (IONS) in Belgium.
2 Several recent studies have shown that it is actually possible to selectively activate nociceptive free nerve endings using a small concentric needle electrode applied against the epidermis. The very focused current generated by the electrode would activate superficial free nerve endings in the epidermis without activating low-threshold mechanoreceptors that are more deeply located (Inui, Tran, Hoshiyama, & Kakigi, 2002; Kaube, Katsarava, Kaufer, Diener, & Ellrich, 2000; Mouraux, Iannetti, & Plaghki, 2010).
3 Recent studies have suggested that mechanical pinprick stimulation using, for example, a thin, flat-tip needle, could be employed to elicit responses predominantly related to the activation of mechanosensitive nociceptors (Iannetti et al., 2013).
4 Other methods have been used to elicit nociceptive ERPs. For example, contact heat-evoked potentials can be recorded using modern contact heat stimulators with very fast heating ramps (Atherton et al., 2007; Gopalakrishnan, Machado, Burgess, & Mosher, 2013). Cooling probes could also be used to elicit ERPs related to the activation of cool- or cold-sensitive afferents. Mechanical pinprick stimulation could be used to record ERPs related specifically to the activation of mechanosensitive nociceptors (Baumgartner, Greffrath, & Treede, 2012). Finally, intraepidermal electrical stimulation could be used to elicit ERPs related to the selective activation of epidermal free nerve endings (Inui et al., 2002; Kaube et al., 2000; Mouraux et al., 2010).
5 In fact, even at the level of the spinal dorsal horn, nociceptive-specific neurons are very sparse (as compared to wide dynamic-range neurons).

References

Allison, T., McCarthy, G., Wood, C. C., Darcey, T. M., Spencer, D. D., & Williamson, P. D. (1989a). Human cortical potentials evoked by stimulation of the median nerve. I. Cytoarchitectonic areas generating short-latency activity. *J Neurophysiol*, 62(3), 694–710.

Allison, T., McCarthy, G., Wood, C. C., Williamson, P. D., & Spencer, D. D. (1989b). Human cortical potentials evoked by stimulation of the median nerve. II. Cytoarchitectonic areas generating long-latency activity. *J Neurophysiol*, 62(3), 711–722.

Andersson, S. A., & Rydenhag, B. (1985). Cortical nociceptive systems. *Philos Trans R Soc Lond B Biol Sci*, 308(1136), 347–359.

Apkarian, A. V., Baliki, M. N., & Farmer, M. A. (2013). Predicting transition to chronic pain. *Curr Opin Neurol*, 26(4), 360–367.

Apkarian, A. V., Bushnell, M. C., Treede, R.-D., & Zubieta, J.-K. (2005). Human brain mechanisms of pain perception and regulation in health and disease. *Eur J Pain*, 9(4), 463–484.

Arthurs, O. J., & Boniface, S. (2002). How well do we understand the neural origins of the fMRI BOLD signal? *Trends Neurosci*, 25(1), 27–31.

Atherton, D. D., Facer, P., Roberts, K. M., Misra, V. P., Chizh, B. A., Bountra, C., & Anand, P. (2007). Use of the novel Contact Heat Evoked Potential Stimulator (CHEPS) for the assessment of small fibre neuropathy: correlations with skin flare responses and intra-epidermal nerve fibre counts. *BMC Neurol*, 7, 21.

Backonja, M., Howland, E. W., Wang, J., Smith, J., Salinsky, M., & Cleeland, C. S. (1991). Tonic changes in alpha power during immersion of the hand in cold water. *Electroencephalogr Clin Neurophysiol*, 79(3), 192–203.

Baier, B., zu Eulenburg, P., Geber, C., Rohde, F., Rolke, R., Maihofner, C., . . . Dieterich, M. (2014). Insula and sensory insular cortex and somatosensory control in patients with insular stroke. *Eur J Pain*, 18(10), 1385–1393.

Baliki, M. N., Chialvo, D. R., Geha, P. Y., Levy, R. M., Harden, R. N., Parrish, T. B., & Apkarian, A. V. (2006). Chronic pain and the emotional brain: specific brain activity associated with spontaneous fluctuations of intensity of chronic back pain. *J Neurosci*, 26(47), 12165–12173.

Baliki, M. N., Petre, B., Torbey, S., Herrmann, K. M., Huang, L., Schnitzer, T. J., . . . Apkarian, A. V. (2012). Corticostriatal functional connectivity predicts transition to chronic back pain. *Nat Neurosci*, 15(8), 1117–1119.

Baumgartner, U., Greffrath, W., & Treede, R. D. (2012). Contact heat and cold, mechanical, electrical and chemical stimuli to elicit small fibre-evoked potentials: merits and limitations for basic science and clinical use. *Neurophysiol Clin*, 42(5), 267–280.

Baumgartner, U., Vogel, H., Ohara, S., Treede, R. D., & Lenz, F. (2011). Dipole source analyses of laser evoked potentials obtained from subdural grid recordings from primary somatic sensory cortex. *J Neurophysiol*, 106(2), 722–730.

Bingel, U., Lorenz, J., Glauche, V., Knab, R., Glascher, J., Weiller, C., & Buchel, C. (2004). Somatotopic organization of human somatosensory cortices for pain: a single trial fMRI study. *Neuroimage*, 23(1), 224–232.

Bingel, U., & Tracey, I. (2008). Imaging CNS modulation of pain in humans. *Physiology (Bethesda)*, 23, 371–380.

Biswal, B., Yetkin, F. Z., Haughton, V. M., & Hyde, J. S. (1995). Functional connectivity in the motor cortex of resting human brain using echo-planar MRI. *Magn Reson Med*, 34(4), 537–541.

Boly, M., Faymonville, M. E., Schnakers, C., Peigneux, P., Lambermont, B., Phillips, C., . . . Laureys, S. (2008). Perception of pain in the minimally conscious state with PET activation: an observational study. *Lancet Neurol*, 7(11), 1013–1020.

Bromm, B., & Treede, R. D. (1984). Nerve fibre discharges, cerebral potentials and sensations induced by CO_2 laser stimulation. *Hum Neurobiol*, 3(1), 33–40.

Bushnell, M. C., & Apkarian, A. V. (2006). Representation of pain in the brain. In S. McMahon & M. Koltzenburg (Eds.), *Wall and Melzack's textbook of pain*, 5th Edition (pp. 267–289). Philadelphia: Elsevier.

Bushnell, M. C., Duncan, G. H., Hofbauer, R. K., Ha, B., Chen, J. I., & Carrier, B. (1999). Pain perception: is there a role for primary somatosensory cortex? *Proc Natl Acad Sci USA*, 96(14), 7705–7709.

Carmon, A., Mor, J., & Goldberg, J. (1976). Evoked cerebral responses to noxious thermal stimuli in humans. *Exp Brain Res*, 25(1), 103–107.

Cauda, F., & Vercelli, A. (2013). How many clusters in the insular cortex? *Cereb Cortex*, 23(11), 2779–2780.

Chapman, C. R., Chen, A. C., Colpitts, Y. M., & Martin, R. W. (1981). Sensory decision theory describes evoked potentials in pain discrimination. *Psychophysiology*, 18(2), 114–120.

Charlesworth, G., Soryal, I., Smith, S., & Sisodiya, S. M. (2009). Acute, localised paroxysmal pain as the initial manifestation of focal seizures: a case report and a brief review of the literature. *Pain*, 141(3), 300–305.

Clark, J. A., Brown, C. A., Jones, A. K., & El-Deredy, W. (2008). Dissociating nociceptive modulation by the duration of pain anticipation from unpredictability in the timing of pain. *Clin Neurophysiol*, 119(12), 2870–2878.

Coghill, R. C., Sang, C. N., Maisog, J. M., & Iadarola, M. J. (1999). Pain intensity processing within the human brain: a bilateral, distributed mechanism. *J Neurophysiol*, 82(4), 1934–1943.

Cole, D. M., Smith, S. M., & Beckmann, C. F. (2010). Advances and pitfalls in the analysis and interpretation of resting-state FMRI data. *Front Syst Neurosci*, 4, 8.

Colon, E., Legrain, V., & Mouraux, A. (2012). Steady-state evoked potentials to study the processing of tactile and nociceptive somatosensory input in the human brain. *Neurophysiol Clin*, 42(5), 315–323.

Colon, E., Legrain, V., & Mouraux, A. (2014). EEG frequency tagging to dissociate the cortical responses to nociceptive and nonnociceptive stimuli. *J Cogn Neurosci*, 26(10), 2262–2274.

Cordes, D., Haughton, V. M., Arfanakis, K., Wendt, G. J., Turski, P. A., Moritz, C. H., . . . Meyerand, M. E. (2000). Mapping functionally related regions of brain with functional connectivity MR imaging. *AJNR Am J Neuroradiol*, 21(9), 1636–1644.

Craig, A. D., Chen, K., Bandy, D., & Reiman, E. M. (2000). Thermosensory activation of insular cortex. *Nat Neurosci*, 3(2), 184–190.

Derbyshire, S. W., Jones, A. K., Gyulai, F., Clark, S., Townsend, D., & Firestone, L. L. (1997). Pain processing during three levels of noxious stimulation produces differential patterns of central activity. *Pain*, 73(3), 431–445.

de Tommaso, M., Navarro, J., Lanzillotti, C., Ricci, K., Buonocunto, F., Livrea, P., & Lancioni, G. E. (2015). Cortical responses to salient nociceptive and not nociceptive stimuli in vegetative and minimal conscious state. *Front Hum Neurosci*, 9, 17.

de Tommaso, M., Navarro, J., Ricci, K., Lorenzo, M., Lanzillotti, C., Colonna, F., . . . Livrea, P. (2013). Pain in prolonged disorders of consciousness: laser evoked potentials findings in patients with vegetative and minimally conscious states. *Brain Inj*, 27(7–8), 962–972.

Dillmann, J., Miltner, W. H., & Weiss, T. (2000). The influence of semantic priming on event-related potentials to painful laser-heat stimuli in humans. *Neurosci Lett*, 284(1–2), 53–56.

DiNuzzo, M. (2014). Isn't functional neuroimaging all about Ca2+ signaling in astrocytes? *J Neurophysiol*, jn 00826.2014.

Dowman, R., Rissacher, D., & Schuckers, S. (2008). EEG indices of tonic pain-related activity in the somatosensory cortices. *Clin Neurophysiol*, 119(5), 1201–1212.

Downar, J., Crawley, A. P., Mikulis, D. J., & Davis, K. D. (2000). A multimodal cortical network for the detection of changes in the sensory environment. *Nat Neurosci*, 3(3), 277–283.

Downar, J., Crawley, A. P., Mikulis, D. J., & Davis, K. D. (2002). A cortical network sensitive to stimulus salience in a neutral behavioral context across multiple sensory modalities. *J Neurophysiol*, 87(1), 615–620.

Dunckley, P., Wise, R. G., Aziz, Q., Painter, D., Brooks, J., Tracey, I., & Chang, L. (2005). Cortical processing of visceral and somatic stimulation: differentiating pain intensity from unpleasantness. *Neuroscience*, 133(2), 533–542.

Feinstein, J. S., Khalsa, S. S., Salomons, T. V., Prkachin, K. M., Frey-Law, L. A., Lee, J. E., . . . Rudrauf, D. (2015). Preserved emotional awareness of pain in a patient with extensive bilateral damage to the insula, anterior cingulate, and amygdala. *Brain Struct Funct*.

Flor, H., Nikolajsen, L., & Staehelin Jensen, T. (2006). Phantom limb pain: a case of maladaptive CNS plasticity? *Nat Rev Neurosci*, 7(11), 873–881.

Forss, N., Raij, T. T., Seppa, M., & Hari, R. (2005). Common cortical network for first and second pain. *Neuroimage*, 24(1), 132–142.

Frot, M., Magnin, M., Mauguiere, F., & Garcia-Larrea, L. (2012). Cortical representation of pain in primary sensory-motor areas (S1/M1) – a study using intracortical recordings in humans. *Hum Brain Mapp*, 34(10), 2655–2668.

Frot, M., & Mauguiere, F. (1999). Timing and spatial distribution of somatosensory responses recorded in the upper bank of the sylvian fissure (SII area) in humans. *Cereb Cortex*, 9(8), 854–863.

Frot, M., & Mauguiere, F. (2003). Dual representation of pain in the operculo-insular cortex in humans. *Brain*, 126(Pt 2), 438–450.

Frot, M., Mauguiere, F., Magnin, M., & Garcia-Larrea, L. (2008). Parallel processing of nociceptive A-delta inputs in SII and midcingulate cortex in humans. *J Neurosci*, 28(4), 944–952.

Frot, M., Rambaud, L., Guenot, M., & Mauguiere, F. (1999). Intracortical recordings of early pain-related CO_2-laser evoked potentials in the human second somatosensory (SII) area. *Clin Neurophysiol*, 110(1), 133–145.

Fukunaga, M., Horovitz, S. G., de Zwart, J. A., van Gelderen, P., Balkin, T. J., Braun, A. R., & Duyn, J. H. (2008). Metabolic origin of BOLD signal fluctuations in the absence of stimuli. *J Cereb Blood Flow Metab*, 28(7), 1377–1387.

Garcia-Larrea, L. (2012). The posterior insular-opercular region and the search of a primary cortex for pain. *Neurophysiol Clin*, 42(5), 299–313.

Garcia-Larrea, L., Frot, M., & Valeriani, M. (2003). Brain generators of laser-evoked potentials: from dipoles to functional significance. *Neurophysiol Clin*, 33(6), 279–292.

Garcia-Larrea, L., & Peyron, R. (2013). Pain matrices and neuropathic pain matrices: a review. *Pain*, 154(Suppl 1), S29–43.

Gopalakrishnan, R., Machado, A. G., Burgess, R. C., & Mosher, J. C. (2013). The use of Contact Heat Evoked Potential Stimulator (CHEPS) in magnetoencephalography for pain research. *J Neurosci Methods*, 220(1), 55–63.

Greenspan, J. D., Lee, R. R., & Lenz, F. A. (1999). Pain sensitivity alterations as a function of lesion location in the parasylvian cortex. *Pain*, 81(3), 273–282.

Greenspan, J. D., & Winfield, J. A. (1992). Reversible pain and tactile deficits associated with a cerebral tumor compressing the posterior insula and parietal operculum. *Pain*, 50(1), 29–39.

Greicius, M. D., Supekar, K., Menon, V., & Dougherty, R. F. (2009). Resting-state functional connectivity reflects structural connectivity in the default mode network. *Cereb Cortex*, 19(1), 72–78.

Gross, J., Schnitzler, A., Timmermann, L., & Ploner, M. (2007). Gamma oscillations in human primary somatosensory cortex reflect pain perception. *PLoS Biol*, 5(5), e133.

Hämäläinen, M., Hari, R., Ilmoniemi, R. J., Knuutila, J., & Lounasmaa, O. V. (1993). Magnetoencephalography: theory, instrumentation, and applications to non-invasive studies of the working human brain. *Reviews of Modern Physics*, 65, 413–497.

Hampson, M., Peterson, B.S., Skudlarski, P., Gatenby, J.C., & Gore, J.C. (2002). Detection of functional connectivity using temporal correlations in MR images. *Hum Brain Mapp*, 15(4), 247–262.

Head, H., & Holmes, G. (1911). Sensory disturbances from cerebral lesions. *Brain*, 34, 102–254.

Hofbauer, R.K., Fiset, P., Plourde, G., Backman, S.B., & Bushnell, M.C. (2004). Dose-dependent effects of propofol on the central processing of thermal pain. *Anesthesiology*, 100(2), 386–394.

Hofbauer, R.K., Rainville, P., Duncan, G.H., & Bushnell, M.C. (2001). Cortical representation of the sensory dimension of pain. *J Neurophysiol*, 86(1), 402–411.

Hu, L., Mouraux, A., Hu, Y., & Iannetti, G.D. (2010). A novel approach for enhancing the signal-to-noise ratio and detecting automatically event-related potentials (ERPs) in single trials. *Neuroimage*, 50(1), 99–111.

Hu, L., Valentini, E., Zhang, Z.G., Liang, M., & Iannetti, G.D. (2014). The primary somatosensory cortex contributes to the latest part of the cortical response elicited by nociceptive somatosensory stimuli in humans. *Neuroimage*, 84, 383–393.

Huang, G., Xiao, P., Hung, Y.S., Iannetti, G.D., Zhang, Z.G., & Hu, L. (2013). A novel approach to predict subjective pain perception from single-trial laser-evoked potentials. *Neuroimage*, 81, 283–293.

Huber, M.T., Bartling, J., Pachur, D., Woikowsky-Biedau, S., & Lautenbacher, S. (2006). EEG responses to tonic heat pain. *Exp Brain Res*, 173(1), 14–24.

Iannetti, G.D., Baumgartner, U., Tracey, I., Treede, R.D., & Magerl, W. (2013). Pinprick-evoked brain potentials: a novel tool to assess central sensitization of nociceptive pathways in humans. *J Neurophysiol*, 110(5), 1107–1116.

Iannetti, G.D., Hughes, N.P., Lee, M.C., & Mouraux, A. (2008). Determinants of laser-evoked EEG responses: pain perception or stimulus saliency? *J Neurophysiol*, 100(2), 815–828.

Iannetti, G.D., & Mouraux, A. (2010). From the neuromatrix to the pain matrix (and back). *Exp Brain Res*, 205(1), 1–12.

Iannetti, G.D., Salomons, T.V., Moayedi, M., Mouraux, A., & Davis, K.D. (2013). Beyond metaphor: contrasting mechanisms of social and physical pain. *Trends Cogn Sci*, 17(8), 371–378.

Iannetti, G.D., Zambreanu, L., Cruccu, G., & Tracey, I. (2005). Operculoinsular cortex encodes pain intensity at the earliest stages of cortical processing as indicated by amplitude of laser-evoked potentials in humans. *Neuroscience*, 131(1), 199–208.

Ingvar, M. (1999). Pain and functional imaging. *Philos Trans R Soc Lond B Biol Sci*, 354(1387), 1347–1358.

Inui, K., Tran, T.D., Hoshiyama, M., & Kakigi, R. (2002). Preferential stimulation of Adelta fibres by intra-epidermal needle electrode in humans. *Pain*, 96(3), 247–252.

Isnard, J., Guenot, M., Sindou, M., & Mauguiere, F. (2004). Clinical manifestations of insular lobe seizures: a stereo-electroencephalographic study. *Epilepsia*, 45(9), 1079–1090.

Jones, A.K., Friston, K., & Frackowiak, R.S. (1992). Localization of responses to pain in human cerebral cortex. *Science*, 255(5041), 215–216.

Kakigi, R., Koyama, S., Hoshiyama, M., Kitamura, Y., Shimojo, M., & Watanabe, S. (1995). Pain-related magnetic fields following painful CO2 laser stimulation in man. *Neurosci Lett*, 192(1), 45–48.

Kakigi, R., Tran, T.D., Qiu, Y., Wang, X., Nguyen, T.B., Inui, K., . . . Hoshiyama, M. (2003). Cerebral responses following stimulation of unmyelinated C-fibres in humans: electro- and magneto-encephalographic study. *Neurosci Res*, 45(3), 255–275.

Kanda, M., Nagamine, T., Ikeda, A., Ohara, S., Kunieda, T., Fujiwara, N., . . . Shibasaki, H. (2000). Primary somatosensory cortex is actively involved in pain processing in human. *Brain Res*, 853(2), 282–289.

Kassubek, J., Juengling, F. D., Els, T., Spreer, J., Herpers, M., Krause, T., . . . Lücking, C. H. (2003). Activation of a residual cortical network during painful stimulation in long-term postanoxic vegetative state: a ^{15}O–H$_2$O PET study. *J Neurol Sci*, 212(1–2), 85–91.

Kaube, H., Katsarava, Z., Kaufer, T., Diener, H., & Ellrich, J. (2000). A new method to increase nociception specificity of the human blink reflex. *Clin Neurophysiol*, 111(3), 413–416.

Kenshalo, D. R., Iwata, K., Sholas, M., & Thomas, D. A. (2000). Response properties and organization of nociceptive neurons in area 1 of monkey primary somatosensory cortex. *J Neurophysiol*, 84(2), 719–729.

Kriegeskorte, N., Goebel, R., & Bandettini, P. (2006). Information-based functional brain mapping. *Proc Natl Acad Sci USA*, 103(10), 3863–3868.

Laureys, S., Faymonville, M. E., Peigneux, P., Damas, P., Lambermont, B., Del Fiore, G., . . . Maquet, P. (2002). Cortical processing of noxious somatosensory stimuli in the persistent vegetative state. *Neuroimage*, 17(2), 732–741.

Lee, M. C., Mouraux, A., & Iannetti, G. D. (2009). Characterizing the cortical activity through which pain emerges from nociception. *J Neurosci*, 29(24), 7909–7916.

Legrain, V., Iannetti, G. D., Plaghki, L., & Mouraux, A. (2010). The pain matrix reloaded: a salience detection system for the body. *Prog Neurobiol*, 93(1), 111–124.

Lenz, F. A., Rios, M., Zirh, A., Chau, D., Krauss, G., & Lesser, R. P. (1998). Painful stimuli evoke potentials recorded over the human anterior cingulate gyrus. *J Neurophysiol*, 79(4), 2231–2234.

Le Pera, D., Svensson, P., Valeriani, M., Watanabe, I., Arendt-Nielsen, L., & Chen, A. C. (2000). Long-lasting effect evoked by tonic muscle pain on parietal EEG activity in humans. *Clin Neurophysiol*, 111(12), 2130–2137.

Liang, M., Mouraux, A., Hu, L., & Iannetti, G. D. (2013a). Primary sensory cortices contain distinguishable spatial patterns of activity for each sense. *Nat Commun*, 4, 1979.

Liang, M., Mouraux, A., & Iannetti, G. D. (2011). Parallel processing of nociceptive and non-nociceptive somatosensory information in the human primary and secondary somatosensory cortices: evidence from dynamic causal modeling of functional magnetic resonance imaging data. *J Neurosci*, 31(24), 8976–8985.

Liang, M., Mouraux, A., & Iannetti, G. D. (2013b). Bypassing primary sensory cortices – a direct thalamocortical pathway for transmitting salient sensory information. *Cereb Cortex*, 23(1), 1–11.

Liu, C. C., Ohara, S., Franaszczuk, P., Zagzoog, N., Gallagher, M., & Lenz, F. A. (2010). Painful stimuli evoke potentials recorded from the medial temporal lobe in humans. *Neuroscience*, 165(4), 1402–1411.

Markl, A., Yu, T., Vogel, D., Muller, F., Kotchoubey, B., & Lang, S. (2013). Brain processing of pain in patients with unresponsive wakefulness syndrome. *Brain Behav*, 3(2), 95–103.

Mayer, E. A., Gupta, A., Kilpatrick, L. A., & Hong, J. Y. (2015). Imaging brain mechanisms in chronic visceral pain. *Pain*, 156 Suppl 1, S50–63.

Miller, G. (2009). Neuroscience. Brain scans of pain raise questions for the law. *Science*, 323(5911), 195.

Mountcastle, V. B. (1957). Modality and topographic properties of single neurons of cat's somatic sensory cortex. *J Neurophysiol*, 20(4), 408–434.

Mountcastle, V. B. (2005). *The sensory hand: neural mechanisms of somatic sensation*. Cambridge: Harvard University Press.

Mouraux, A., Diukova, A., Lee, M.C., Wise, R.G., & Iannetti, G.D. (2011a). A multisensory investigation of the functional significance of the "pain matrix." *Neuroimage*, 54(3), 2237–2249.

Mouraux, A., Gille, M., Dorban, S., & Peeters, A. (2002). Cortical venous thrombosis after lumbar puncture. *J Neurol*, 249(9), 1313–1315.

Mouraux, A., Guerit, J.M., & Plaghki, L. (2003). Non-phase locked electroencephalogram (EEG) responses to CO2 laser skin stimulations may reflect central interactions between A partial partial differential- and C-fibre afferent volleys. *Clin Neurophysiol*, 114(4), 710–722.

Mouraux, A., Guerit, J.M., & Plaghki, L. (2004). Refractoriness cannot explain why C-fibre laser-evoked brain potentials are recorded only if concomitant Adelta-fibre activation is avoided. *Pain*, 112(1–2), 16–26.

Mouraux, A., & Iannetti, G.D. (2008). Across-trial averaging of event-related EEG responses and beyond. *Magn Reson Imaging*, 26(7), 1041–1054.

Mouraux, A., & Iannetti, G.D. (2009). Nociceptive laser-evoked brain potentials do not reflect nociceptive-specific neural activity. *J Neurophysiol*, 101(6), 3258–3269.

Mouraux, A., Iannetti, G.D., Colon, E., Nozaradan, S., Legrain, V., & Plaghki, L. (2011b). Nociceptive steady-state evoked potentials elicited by rapid periodic thermal stimulation of cutaneous nociceptors. *J Neurosci*, 31(16), 6079–6087.

Mouraux, A., Iannetti, G.D., & Plaghki, L. (2010). Low intensity intra-epidermal electrical stimulation can activate Adelta-nociceptors selectively. *Pain*, 150(1), 199–207.

Mouraux, A., & Plaghki, L. (2007). Cortical interactions and integration of nociceptive and non-nociceptive somatosensory inputs in humans. *Neuroscience*, 150(1), 72–81.

Mur, M., Bandettini, P.A., & Kriegeskorte, N. (2009). Revealing representational content with pattern-information fMRI – an introductory guide. *Soc Cogn Affect Neurosci*, 4(1), 101–109.

Nunez, P.L., & Srinivasan, R. (2006). *Electric fields of the brain: the neurophysics of EEG* (2nd Edition). New York: Oxford University Press.

Ohara, S., Crone, N.E., Weiss, N., Treede, R.D., & Lenz, F.A. (2004). Cutaneous painful laser stimuli evoke responses recorded directly from primary somatosensory cortex in awake humans. *J Neurophysiol*, 91(6), 2734–2746.

Ostrowsky, K., Magnin, M., Ryvlin, P., Isnard, J., Guenot, M., & Mauguiere, F. (2002). Representation of pain and somatic sensation in the human insula: a study of responses to direct electrical cortical stimulation. *Cereb Cortex*, 12(4), 376–385.

Peng, W., Hu, L., Zhang, Z., & Hu, Y. (2014). Changes of spontaneous oscillatory activity to tonic heat pain. *PLoS One*, 9(3), e91052.

Peyron, R., Frot, M., Schneider, F., Garcia-Larrea, L., Mertens, P., Barral, F.G., . . . Mauguiere, F. (2002). Role of operculoinsular cortices in human pain processing: converging evidence from PET, fMRI, dipole modeling, and intracerebral recordings of evoked potentials. *Neuroimage*, 17(3), 1336–1346.

Peyron, R., Laurent, B., & Garcia-Larrea, L. (2000). Functional imaging of brain responses to pain: a review and meta-analysis (2000). *Neurophysiol Clin*, 30(5), 263–288.

Plaghki, L., & Mouraux, A. (2002). Brain responses to signals ascending through C-fibres. In K. Hirata (Ed.), *International Congress Series* (Vol. 1232, pp. 181–192). Amsterdam: Elsevier.

Plaghki, L., & Mouraux, A. (2003). How do we selectively activate skin nociceptors with a high power infrared laser? Physiology and biophysics of laser stimulation. *Neurophysiol Clin*, 33(6), 269–277.

Plaghki, L., & Mouraux, A. (2005). EEG and laser stimulation as tools for pain research. *Curr Opin Investig Drugs*, 6(1), 58–64.

Ploner, M., Gross, J., Timmermann, L., Pollok, B., & Schnitzler, A. (2006). Pain suppresses spontaneous brain rhythms. *Cerebral cortex*, 16(4), 537–540.

Ploner, M., Schmitz, F., Freund, H. J., & Schnitzler, A. (1999). Parallel activation of primary and secondary somatosensory cortices in human pain processing. *J Neurophysiol*, 81(6), 3100–3104.

Ploner, M., Schoffelen, J. M., Schnitzler, A., & Gross, J. (2009). Functional integration within the human pain system as revealed by Granger causality. *Hum Brain Mapp*, 30(12), 4025–4032.

Poldrack, R. A. (2006). Can cognitive processes be inferred from neuroimaging data? *Trends Cogn Sci*, 10(2), 59–63.

Porro, C. A. (2003). Functional imaging and pain: behavior, perception, and modulation. *Neuroscientist*, 9(5), 354–369.

Qiu, Y., Inui, K., Wang, X., Nguyen, B. T., Tran, T. D., & Kakigi, R. (2004). Effects of distraction on magnetoencephalographic responses ascending through C-fibres in humans. *Clin Neurophysiol*, 115(3), 636–646.

Rainville, P. (2002). Brain mechanisms of pain affect and pain modulation. *Curr Opin Neurobiol*, 12(2), 195–204.

Rainville, P., Duncan, G. H., Price, D. D., Carrier, B., & Bushnell, M. C. (1997). Pain affect encoded in human anterior cingulate but not somatosensory cortex. *Science*, 277(5328), 968–971.

Regan, D. (1989). *Human brain electrophysiology: evoked potentials and evoked magnetic fields in science and medicine*. New York: Elsevier.

Ringler, R., Greiner, M., Kohlloeffel, L., Handwerker, H. O., & Forster, C. (2003). BOLD effects in different areas of the cerebral cortex during painful mechanical stimulation. *Pain*, 105(3), 445–453.

Schulz, E., May, E. S., Postorino, M., Tiemann, L., Nickel, M. M., Witkovsky, V., . . . Ploner, M. (2015). *Prefrontal gamma oscillations encode tonic pain in humans*. Cereb Cortex, Epub ahead of print.

Schweinhardt, P., Bountra, C., & Tracey, I. (2006). Pharmacological FMRI in the development of new analgesic compounds. *NMR Biomed*, 19(6), 702–711.

Seeley, W. W., Menon, V., Schatzberg, A. F., Keller, J., Glover, G. H., Kenna, H., . . . Greicius, M. D. (2007). Dissociable intrinsic connectivity networks for salience processing and executive control. *J Neurosci*, 27(9), 2349–2356.

Segerdahl, A. R., Mezue, M., Okell, T. W., Farrar, J. T., & Tracey, I. (2015). The dorsal posterior insula subserves a fundamental role in human pain. *Nat Neurosci*, 18(4), 499–500.

Sherrington, R. (1906). *The integrative action of the nervous system*. New Haven: Yale University Press.

Stowell, H. (1984). Event related brain potentials and human pain: a first objective overview. *Int J Psychophysiol*, 1(2), 137–151.

Talbot, J. D., Marrett, S., Evans, A. C., Meyer, E., Bushnell, M. C., & Duncan, G. H. (1991). Multiple representations of pain in human cerebral cortex. *Science*, 251(4999), 1355–1358.

Tolle, T. R., Kaufmann, T., Siessmeier, T., Lautenbacher, S., Berthele, A., Munz, F., . . . Bartenstein, P. (1999). Region-specific encoding of sensory and affective components of pain in the human brain: a positron emission tomography correlation analysis. *Ann Neurol*, 45(1), 40–47.

Tommerdahl, M., Delemos, K. A., Vierck, C. J., Jr., Favorov, O. V., & Whitsel, B. L. (1996). Anterior parietal cortical response to tactile and skin-heating stimuli applied to the same skin site. *J Neurophysiol*, 75(6), 2662–2670.

Tracey, I., & Mantyh, P. W. (2007). The cerebral signature for pain perception and its modulation. *Neuron*, 55(3), 377–391.

Tran, T.D., Inui, K., Hoshiyama, M., Lam, K., Qiu, Y., & Kakigi, R. (2002). Cerebral activation by the signals ascending through unmyelinated C-fibres in humans: a magneto-encephalographic study. *Neuroscience*, 113(2), 375–386.

Treede, R.D., Kenshalo, D.R., Gracely, R.H., & Jones, A.K. (1999). The cortical representation of pain. *Pain*, 79(2–3), 105–111.

Treede, R.D., Kief, S., Holzer, T., & Bromm, B. (1988). Late somatosensory evoked cerebral potentials in response to cutaneous heat stimuli. *Electroencephalogr Clin Neurophysiol*, 70(5), 429–441.

Treede, R.D., Meier, W., Kunze, K., & Bromm, B. (1988). Ultralate cerebral potentials as correlates of delayed pain perception: observation in a case of neurosyphilis. *J Neurol Neurosurg Psychiatry*, 51(10), 1330–1333.

Valentini, E., Hu, L., Chakrabarti, B., Hu, Y., Aglioti, S.M., & Iannetti, G.D. (2012). The primary somatosensory cortex largely contributes to the early part of the cortical response elicited by nociceptive stimuli. *Neuroimage*, 59(2), 1571–1581.

Valeriani, M., Restuccia, D., Le Pera, D., De Armas, L., Maiese, T., & Tonali, P. (2002). Attention-related modifications of ultra-late CO(2) laser evoked potentials to human trigeminal nerve stimulation. *Neurosci Lett*, 329(3), 329–333.

Wager, T.D., Atlas, L.Y., Lindquist, M.A., Roy, M., Woo, C.W., & Kross, E. (2013). An fMRI-based neurologic signature of physical pain. *N Engl J Med*, 368(15), 1388–1397.

Wall, P.D. (1995). Independent mechanisms converge on pain. *Nat Med*, 1(8), 740–741.

Wall, P.D., McMahon, S.B., & Koltzenburg, M. (2006). *Wall and Melzack's textbook of pain* (5th Edition). Philadelphia: Elsevier.

Whitsel, B.L., Favorov, O.V., Li, Y., Quibrera, M., & Tommerdahl, M. (2009). Area 3a neuron response to skin nociceptor afferent drive. *Cereb Cortex*, 19(2), 349–366.

Xu, X., Kanda, M., Shindo, K., Fujiwara, N., Nagamine, T., Ikeda, A., . . . Kaji, R. (1995). Pain-related somatosensory evoked potentials following CO2 laser stimulation of foot in man. *Electroencephalogr Clin Neurophysiol*, 96(1), 12–23.

Yarkoni, T., Poldrack, R.A., Nichols, T.E., Van Essen, D.C., & Wager, T.D. (2011). Large-scale automated synthesis of human functional neuroimaging data. *Nat Methods*, 8(8), 665–670.

Young, G.B., & Blume, W.T. (1983). Painful epileptic seizures. *Brain*, 106(Pt 3), 537–554.

Zhang, Z.G., Hu, L., Hung, Y.S., Mouraux, A., & Iannetti, G.D. (2012). Gamma-band oscillations in the primary somatosensory cortex – a direct and obligatory correlate of subjective pain intensity. *J Neurosci*, 32(22), 7429–7438.

zu Eulenburg, P., Baumgartner, U., Treede, R.D., & Dieterich, M. (2013). Interoceptive and multimodal functions of the operculo-insular cortex: tactile, nociceptive and vestibular representations. *Neuroimage*, 83, 75–86.

3 Behavioral assessment of pain in disorders of consciousness

Clinical and ethical issues

Nathan D. Zasler,[1] *Anne T. O'Brien,*[2] *and Caroline Schnakers*[3]

Abbreviations

ACC	anterior cingulate cortex
DOC	disorders of consciousness
HO	heterotopic ossification
MCS	minimally conscious state
NCS (-R)	Nociception Coma Scale (-Revised)
PET	positron emission tomography
S1	primary somatosensory cortex
S2	secondary somatosensory cortex
VS/UWS	vegetative state/unresponsive wakefulness syndrome

Introduction

Pain is defined as "an unpleasant sensory and emotional experience associated with real or potential tissue damage" (IASP, 1994), whereas nociception is described as "an actually or potentially tissue damaging event transduced and encoded by nociceptors" (Loeser, Treede, 2008). Nociception hence refers to the basic processing of a noxious stimulus. It is necessary to pain perception but it will not always lead to a conscious experience (Loeser, Treede, 2008). In contrast, pain is a conscious first-person experience that has to be reported, verbally or non-verbally, to be correctly assessed.

The challenge with noncommunicative patients is how to establish if they are in fact in pain. Patients with severe brain injury are often unable to communicate their feelings, including pain and suffering experiences. According to the IASP (International Association for the Study of Pain), the inability to communicate verbally does not exclude the possibility that an individual is experiencing pain and needs appropriate pain-relieving treatment (IASP, 1994). The aforementioned position emphasizes the need for better ways to assess pain perception and suffering in those who are severely impaired following brain injury. Progress in intensive care and neuroimaging has positively impacted the number of patients recovering from coma. A growing number of recent studies have investigated pain perception and its assessment in patients who are in states of disordered consciousness following severe brain injury. This chapter will explain our current knowledge of residual pain perception in conscious patients (i.e., minimally conscious state [MCS]) (Giacino et al., 2002) versus unconscious patients (i.e., vegetative state/unresponsive wakefulness syndrome [VS/UWS]) (Jennett, Plum, 1972); how assessment and management of pain is possible in such a population; and the ethical challenges related to this important clinical issue.

Neuroimaging data

MCS versus VS/UWS

In patients diagnosed as being in a MCS, Boly et al. reported brain activation similar to that seen in controls in response to noxious stimuli encompassing not only the midbrain, the thalamus, and the primary somatosensory cortex (S1), but also the secondary somatosensory (S2) and insular cortex, the posterior parietal, and the posterior part of the anterior cingulate cortex (ACC) (Boly et al., 2008). The activation of these areas (and particularly the ACC and insula) suggests that patients in a MCS may perceive the unpleasant aspect of painful stimuli (Bingel et al., 2002; Shackman et al., 2011, see also Chapter 2 for further discussion about pain processing in humans) and so implies the potential to suffer. Moreover, intact connectivity between primary and associative cortices has also been observed in these patients, suggesting the existence of an integrated and distributed neural processing that makes the existence of conscious pain perception in this population plausible (see Figure 3.1).

In patients diagnosed as being in a VS/UWS, Laureys et al. (2002) investigated central processing of noxious stimuli by using H_2O positron emission tomography (PET) imaging in post-comatose patients (Laureys et al., 2002) (see Figure 3.1). An increase of metabolism was observed in midbrain, contralateral thalamus, and S1 in response to an electrical stimulation applied to the median nerve of the wrist in a group of 15 patients in a VS/UWS. The activated S1 was functionally disconnected from S2, bilateral posterior parietal, premotor, polysensory superior temporal, and prefrontal cortices as compared to 15 healthy controls. Furthermore, recent findings suggest that long-distance connectivity (e.g., between frontal and temporal areas) is more impaired than short-distance connectivity (e.g., in areas within the temporal gyrus) in VS/UWS, which may be crucial for integrative brain processing leading to consciousness (Boly et al., 2011). There is apparently a disruption in signal processing not only at the cortical level but also in the signal transmission from the subcortical to the cortical level. A reemergence of functional connectivity between the thalamus and associative areas has been previously found in patients recovering from the VS/UWS (Laureys et al., 2000). This observation is particularly important as the thalamus constitutes a relay in transmitting sensory/pain signals from subcortical to cortical areas and has a key role in conscious processing (Zasler, Martelli, Nicholson, 2013). In fact, Lutkenhoff et al. (2013) have recently shown that the extent of atrophy observed in the anterior thalamic nucleus predicts recovery of consciousness at six months post-injury. These results suggest the presence of impaired and disconnected residual brain activity in VS/UWS patients, reducing the probability that painful stimuli are experienced in an integrated and conscious manner.

Really, no pain?

It is important to stress that, despite these neuroimaging studies, it is still unclear whether all patients in a VS/UWS are unable to feel pain and/or if they suffer due to pain. Kassubek et al. (2003) performed a H_2O PET scan when administering an electrical noxious stimulus in seven post-anoxic patients in a VS/UWS. A group analysis revealed a pain-induced activation in S1, but also in S2 and in the cingulate cortex, which is involved in the affective pain network. More recently, de Tommaso et al. (2013) used nociceptive specific laser evoked potentials known to be related to pain generators, such as the ACC, and have reported a response (with a longer latency) in three patients in a VS/UWS. Two other studies reported an activation of the affective pain network (i.e., ACC and insula) in 30% of patients in a VS/UWS in response to noxious stimulation, as well as pain cries (Markl et al., 2013; Yu et al., 2013) In Figure 3.1, Panel A illustrates, in yellow/red, brain regions activated during noxious stimulation in healthy controls, in patients in a minimally conscious state (MCS), and in a vegetative state/unresponsive wakefulness syndrome (VS/UWS) (Boly et al., 2008; Laureys et al., 2002). Panel B illustrates the unusual activation of the secondary somatosensory area in response to noxious stimulation in one patient diagnosed as being in a VS/UWS (Markl et al., 2013). Nevertheless Yu et al., (2013) also showed, consistent with previous findings, that the connectivity within the whole pain network was significantly decreased in patients in a VS/UWS as compared to patients in a MCS (Kotchoubey et al., 2013). Even though this suggests an altered perception in patients in a VS/UWS, the activation of the affective pain network might denote the presence of residual pain perception in some of those patients. As a minority of patients behaviorally diagnosed as being in a VS/UWS have previously shown brain activation in response to active cognitive tasks (Monti et al., 2010; Schnakers, Perrin, Schabus et al., 2009; Cruse et al., 2011), it is also plausible to assume that a percentage of patients who do not show behavioral signs of consciousness may be able to perceive external stimuli, such as pain. Finally, voluntary and reflexive behaviors can be difficult to distinguish and subtle signs of consciousness can be missed due to fluctuations in vigilance or motor/verbal impairments (i.e., around 40% of patients diagnosed as being in a VS/UWS are misdiagnosed and are in fact conscious) (Schnakers, Vanhaudenhuyse, Giacino et al., 2009). This underlines the importance of considering the potential experience of pain in all patients with disorders of consciousness (DOC) and of developing tools to appropriately assess and treat pain in those patients (Schnakers, Zasler, 2007). (Refer to Figure 3.1 in Colour Plate Section.)

Behavioral assessment of pain

Pain management in patients with DOC remains challenging since the assessment is limited by the absence of communication. Several scales have been developed and validated to detect pain in noncommunicative patients such as newborns (Hummel, van Dijk, 2006) or patients with dementia (American Geriatrics Society, 2002). However, until recently, no scale had been developed to assess pain in patients with DOC. Patients in a VS/UWS can demonstrate responses, such as grimaces, cries, tachycardia, or tachypnea. These responses may follow pathological activation of subcortical pathways in reflexive response to pain but may also be unrelated to painful stimuli (The Multi-Society Task Force on PVS, 1994). It is therefore necessary to develop sensitive standardized tools to accurately assess responses related to nociception and pain in this population.

The Nociception Coma Scale

Recently, a new scale was developed to assess nociception and pain in patients with DOC – the Nociception Coma Scale (NCS) Schnakers et al., Pain 2010 (NCSR). The term "nociception" was chosen for two reasons. First, the NCS aims to assess patients in both a VS/UWS and in a MCS and is therefore assessing responses underlying both low-level brain processing related to nociception (as observed in a majority of patients in a VS/UWS) and high-level brain processing related to pain (as observed in patients in a MCS). Second, as pain is a subjective experience, it is difficult to use the term "pain" when no self-report is available.

The first version of the NCS (Schnakers et al., 2010) was based on preexisting pain scales developed for newborns and noncommunicative patients with advanced dementia (American Geriatrics Society, 2002; Hummel, van Dijk, 2006). It consisted of four subscales assessing motor, verbal, and visual responses to noxious stimuli as well as facial expression. Its total score ranged from zero to 12. Initially, breathing responses were also assessed but they were later discarded due to the difficulty of reliably assessing breathing patterns in patients not benefiting from respiratory monitoring devices (which is often the case in a subacute setting) (Schnakers et al., 2010). Previous studies have also shown that physiological parameters seem insufficiently sensitive for pain assessment (Herr et al., 2011), as pain was found to be unreliably related to self-reports (Gelinas, Arbour, 2009; Gelinas, Johnston, 2007) and to fluctuate similarly in response to both non-noxious or noxious stimulation (Young et al., 2006). Stress, medication, and medical complications, but also brain lesions affecting autonomic functions, may also influence these parameters and bias the assessment (Buttner, Finke, 2000; Herr, Garand, 2001).

The NCS has been validated in patients from intensive care, neurology/neurosurgery units, rehabilitation centers, and nursing homes. In a first study including 48 patients (28 VS/UWS and 20 MCS; age range 20–82 years; 17 of traumatic etiology), behavioral responses to a noxious stimulus (i.e., nail bed pressure) were scored by two raters using the NCS and four other scales previously validated for noncommunicative patients (e.g., the Pain Assessment In Advanced Dementia Scale; Warden et al., 2003). Results demonstrated good inter-rater reliability and good concurrent validity for the NCS total scores and subscores. Those good psychometric properties have also been replicated in other studies investigating the validity and reliability of the translated versions of the scale (i.e., in Italian and in Dutch) (Sattin et al., 2013; Vink et al., 2014). Compared to the other pain scales, the NCS showed a broader score range and a better sensitivity to clinical diagnosis. Patients in a VS/UWS showed lower scores than those in a MCS, which suggests that the NCS is particularly relevant for the evaluation of pain in patients with DOC. Although those results support the good psychometric properties of the scale, they do not ensure that the observed behavioral changes were actually specific to the noxious stimulus administered as the changes may also occur spontaneously or in response to non-noxious stimuli.

A second study assessing 64 patients (27 VS/UWS and 37 MCS; age range 20–82 years; 22 of traumatic etiology) was therefore performed in order to compare NCS scores observed at rest, in response to a non-noxious stimulus (i.e., tap on the shoulders), and in response to a noxious stimulus (i.e., nail bed pressure). Results showed that NCS total scores, as well as motor, verbal, and facial subscores, were significantly higher in response to a noxious stimulus than the scores at rest or in response to a non-noxious stimulus, reflecting the good sensitivity of the scale. However, no difference could be observed between noxious and non-noxious conditions for the visual subscores, which suggests that this subscale was not specific to nociception. The authors therefore decided to propose a new version of the scale excluding the visual subscale – the Nociception Coma Scale – Revised (NCS-R) (Chatelle et al., 2012) (see Table 3.1).

Finally, a recent neuroimaging study has investigated whether the NCS-R is related to brain areas involved in the so-called pain matrix (Chatelle, Thibaut,

Table 3.1 The Nociception Coma Scale-Revised (NCS-R)

MOTOR RESPONSES
 3—Localization to painful stimulation
 2—Flexion withdrawal
 1—Abnormal posturing
 0—None/Flaccid

VERBAL RESPONSES
 3—Verbalization (intelligible)
 2—Vocalization
 1—Groaning
 0—None

FACIAL RESPONSES
 3—Cry
 2—Grimace
 1—Oral reflexive movement/Startle response
 0—None

Bruno et al., 2014). Using 18-Fluoro-deoxyglucose PET scan, a significant correlation was found between NCS-R total scores and brain metabolism in the ACC. Those results suggest that the NCS-R at least partially correlates with cortical pain processing and hence may constitute an appropriate behavioral tool to assess, monitor, and treat nociception and pain in non-communicative patients with DOC.

A case report on pain management

A 23-year-old female pedestrian was struck by a motor vehicle. She sustained a traumatic brain injury with neuroimaging findings showing open skull fracture, depressed frontal bone, and subdural hematoma in the left frontal area. She was admitted to the rehabilitation hospital five weeks after injury. She was diagnosed as being in a VS/UWS according to the Coma Recovery Scale-Revised (Giacino et al., 2004) with a total score of 4/23 (i.e., behaviorally demonstrating flexion withdrawal, oral reflexive movement, and eye opening with stimulation). Pain was evaluated daily using the NCS-R. Scores of zero (indicating no pain behaviors) were observed during her treatment sessions. Two weeks after admission to the rehabilitation center, the NCS-R scores suddenly increased. It was noted that, when stretching her right hip into flexion during physical therapy sessions, she had abnormal flexion, tongue pumping, and chewing movements of the mouth. These behaviors were observed only when mobilizing the patient in this manner and not on other occasions, suggesting that these behaviors were linked to this particular stimulation. Following a discussion with her medical doctor about these findings, an X-ray of her right hip was ordered. Imaging showed heterotopic ossification (HO) adjacent to the right lesser trochanter and inferior to the right femoral head. The plan of care changed to schedule pain medication prior to lower extremity stretching. Physical therapy and pain rating using the NCS-R continued daily, in addition to weekly range of motion measurements to evaluate the clinical status of the HO that had developed.

As we see in the case described above, the NCS-R may constitute a helpful instrument for monitoring pain behavior on a daily basis and should be administered to all patients who are in a VS/UWS or in a MCS – and especially to those who present a documented potential pain (e.g., as here, polytraumatic injuries). A sudden increase in the NCS-R total score during hospitalization independent of an improvement in the level of consciousness will alert the clinician of the potential presence of pain. Additional investigations may then be performed to identify its origin/location (e.g., as here, by using mobilization during physical therapy sessions and by ordering an X-ray). Behavioral signs of pain at rest (e.g., grimaces or cries) can be taken into consideration. However, those responses could be unrelated to pain (e.g., pathological activation of subcortical areas leading to constant but not appropriate cries) (The Multi-Society Task Force on PVS, 1994) and therefore should be replicated in a pain-related condition (i.e., mobilization/palpation). The NCS-R should be scored at rest in order to observe the spontaneous responses presented by the patient (assessed with eyes opened) for at least one minute before starting potentially painful care and/or stimulation. Behavioral responses observed during the care and/or stimulation are then scored with the NCS-R. The highest score obtained for each subscale is summed to obtain the total score.

Particular attention should be given to patients with spasticity, as it is a frequent condition in long-lasting DOC. A recent study showed that 89% of patients who were in either a chronic VS/UWS or a MCS (N=65) demonstrated signs of spasticity (Modified Ashworth Scale, MAS ≥ 1), including 60% who showed severe spasticity (MAS ≥ 3). The authors found that the severity of spasticity is correlated to pain, as measured by the NCS-R, which highlights the importance of pain management in non-communicative patients with severe brain injury (Thibaut et al., 2014). In cases where there is a documented cause of potential pain, the NCS-R should be administered both before and after treatment. It is essential to simultaneously assess the patient's level of consciousness in order to avoid overmedication. Indeed, it is likely that the administration of narcotic or other sedating analgesics will decrease not only the presence of pain behaviors but also the presence of signs of consciousness as those medications may have an impact on alertness and vigilance in patients who already show deficits in those domains (Lanzillo et al., 2014). Therefore, it is critical to monitor the impact of the administered treatment in order to avoid under- or over-medication, and to revise such treatment regularly if clinically indicated.

Pain ethics in persons with disorders of consciousness

The topic of pain ethics in persons with DOC is a relatively new area of bio-ethics, as the topic of pain has received little attention in the scientific literature until relatively recently (Schnakers, Zasler, 2007). A number of salient ethical issues are intimately intertwined with the issue of pain in persons with DOC. Some of these ethical challenges have solutions driven by logical deductive reasoning, some by general consensus, and some, albeit few, by science. A number of the ethical challenges in the context of DOC-related pain have no simple answers and polar viewpoints abound. Unfortunately, the topic of pain in DOC, and more specifically the ethical quagmire that it presents, has been relatively ignored in recent relevant major publications (Posner, et al., 2007; Laureys, Tononi, 2009); however, it is clearly a topic of importance for further discussion and debate that should be included in any treatise on the topic of severe brain injury and DOC.

Factors impacting practice

In the context of this discussion, it is important to understand how many different factors impact ethics of practice in how persons with DOC are evaluated and treated, including for pain disorders. These factors include cultural background (of both the treating professionals and the patient/family/surrogate), professional training and experience with patients with DOC, politico-legal and health-care systems, and moral and religious beliefs. For example, traditional Judeo-Christian views advocate for preservation of life even in the presence of pain and/or suffering when there is no imminent demise. In Islamic law and teachings, end-of-life suffering is seen as a way to purify sins. All three of the aforementioned religions generally take the perspective that life must be preserved regardless of the state of the individual, pain or no pain, suffering or no suffering, with rare exceptions, as life is sacred and a gift of God and only to be ended by God (Pew Research Religion & Public Life Project, 2013).

Given that the views of practitioners working with this patient group are often polar from how they themselves would like to be cared for if they were in the same situation, it certainly becomes an ethical challenge for many a clinician to separate personal values from the science of DOC assessment and care (Demertzi, et al., 2009; Demertzi, et al., 2014). There is very little published data exploring how the aforementioned factors ultimately impact the accuracy of overall assessment (including that of pain), and/or the aggressiveness of care (or lack thereof) for the patient with DOC, including care related to pain conditions.

Some have also suggested the need to explore the social aspects of ethics in DOC, in the context of what has been termed "pragmatic neuroethics," in an attempt to promote nonreductionistic understandings of the ethical dilemmas raised by the care of patients with DOC (Racine, 2013). Pragmatic neuroethics can certainly also be applied to addressing issues of pain and suffering.

The ethical burden of pain and suffering

When dealing with pain and suffering, both in general and specifically in persons with DOC, it is of paramount importance to consider patient autonomy, competency issues including assignment of surrogates, nonmaleficence, beneficence, and justice (Banja, Fins, 2013). In the absence of a more complete understanding of the neural correlates of pain and suffering in persons with DOC, we are all faced with the ethical challenge of how ultimately to consolidate behavioral and instrumental observations to develop a medically probable opinion on whether a given individual is consciously aware of pain (as opposed to demonstrating reflexive responses to pain) and, maybe even more importantly, whether that person suffers due to the pain experienced (Boly, Faymonville, et al., 2005). As noted by Bernat, "no one can directly experience the conscious awareness of another person, thus a clinician's determination of a patient's unawareness is by necessity inferential" (Bernat, 2009).

Pain constitutes a conscious experience with physical and psychological components of nociception and suffering. There remains debate about how much of the pain neuromatrix must be functional in order for the patient to experience pain and ultimately to suffer, with suffering being related to the cognitive–evaluative and motivational–affective aspects of pain processing. That being said, we do not know if structures that normally participate in pain and suffering responses in the healthy brain are all necessary for experiencing pain and suffering in the person with an injured brain or what differences there might be in the qualitative experience of pain, or suffering in the latter scenario. There also remains debate about whether the so-called pain neural matrix is truly pain specific, as opposed to being an epiphenomena (Pistoia, et al., 2013).

The question of whether pain can be experienced at a subcortical level is part of these debates (Shewmon, 2004; Demertzi, Laureys, et al., 2011; for additional information about pain processing, see Chapter 2).

Examination ethics and DOC pain

Given the diagnostic challenges presented by these patients, it is of utmost importance for us, as clinicians, to optimize examination conditions so that patients have every opportunity to demonstrate awareness. We do this through use of standardized examination techniques (i.e., making sure there is adequate arousal, examining lying down and sitting up, and assessing when off sedating medications, among other measures; see also Chapter 4) with standardized scoring scales for responses to stimuli, including pain assessment measures relevant to persons in DOC Schnakers et al., Pain 2010 (NCSR), as well as through optimizing medical stability and pharmacologic regimens as the latter might otherwise confound interpretation of exam findings.

The absence of behavioral markers of pain experience on examination cannot be inferred to mean that an individual does not consciously perceive pain and/ or suffer as a consequence. Similarly, certain behavioral responses may cause less experienced and knowledgeable practitioners to conclude that there is conscious perception of pain and/or suffering when in fact there is not. Based on our current understanding, an individual's state of disordered consciousness may not even be predictive, in and of itself, of the individual's ability to feel pain; that is, there is some evidence that persons in a VS/UWS may show pain responses (Chatelle, Thibaut, Bruno, et al., 2014). We do not know how much residual cognition (e.g., memory) is necessary to enable suffering in persons in MCS. There has been a shift to relying more on instrumental assessments via such modalities as neuroimaging and electrophysiological testing (i.e., auditory mismatch negativity, somatosensory evoked potentials) than on the behavioral assessment methodologies as advocated by Giacino and others (Giacino, et al., 2013; Farisco, Petrini, 2014) that have been historically relied upon and that remain the "gold standard" (Bodart, et al., 2013). Others have even advocated for use of more highly relevant stimuli in the context of multimodal pain assessment in DOC to confirm cortical arousal to pain salience (de Tommaso, et al., 2013). Ultimately, correct diagnosis of the state of DOC and appropriate behavioral, as well as instrumental, assessment are paramount to beginning the necessary discussion of whether a given individual may have the potential to experience pain and suffer.

How the advances in instrumental technology, including functional neuroimaging and electrophysiological assessment, have actually, in practical terms, contributed to the assessment and treatment of pain and suffering in persons with DOC is still an unanswered question. Playing devil's advocate, we do not know for certain whether all aspects of central pain processing are being "tapped" by such advances, which leads to the quandary of whether we can ever be certain that someone in a state of disordered consciousness really does not feel pain or have the ability to suffer due to pain (Friedrich, 2013).

It is also clearly important to appreciate the fact that the experience of pain and suffering in persons with DOC likely occurs along a continuum from absent, to partial, to completely normal – and that may also change, over time, in either direction. More specifically, we know that functional recovery occurs following traumatic brain injury and DOC for at least five years, if not more (Nakase-Richardson, Whyte, et al., 2012). This knowledge brings into question the common practice of transitioning care from rehabilitation settings early after injury if the patient remains in a state of disordered consciousness and relegating care beyond that point to practitioners in nursing home settings without allocation for providing specialized follow-up for reassessment at periodic intervals. It is also important to acknowledge that patients with severe brain injury and resultant DOC may also regress functionally and neurologically over time and therefore are prone to be at higher risk of developing new pain generators compared to those who improve over time.

Health professional ethical obligations

What are our obligations as health professionals to ensure that we are doing all we can to adequately assess, as well as ameliorate, pain and suffering in persons with DOC? Is it ethically relevant to determine if someone is suffering or not in the context of clinical decision-making in this population? Does it matter? And if so, why? How important is amelioration of pain for the patient beyond quality of life? Can it make a difference in other areas, such as in level of function and/ or consciousness (Lanzillo, et al., 2014; Pistoia, et al., 2015)?

For health-care practitioners working with persons with DOC and pain, it would hopefully be apparent that pain alleviation is a human right; yet, surprisingly, mainstream medical organizations generally do not consider pain management as a duty of the physician. Some have even argued that there are adverse potential consequences to pursuing pain management, in general, as a fundamental right of all patients since it may place other factors – such as politics, third party payers, and others – in the middle of the physician-patient relationship (Hall, Boswell, 2009). Yet others have taken a strongly polar position on this issue. The Institute of Medicine, in their document entitled "Relieving Pain in America: A Blueprint for Transforming Prevention, Care, Education and Research." noted that "Effective pain management is a moral imperative, a professional responsibility, and the duty of people in the healing professions" (IOM, 2011). The International Association for the Study of Pain published the "Declaration that Access to Pain Management is a Fundamental Human Right" and further noted that it is critical to recognize the intrinsic dignity of all persons and the fact that withholding pain treatment is profoundly wrong and leads to unnecessary suffering, which is harmful. The document goes on to note that there must be an international recognition of three pain-related rights including:

> The right of all people to have access to pain management without discrimination; the right of people in pain to acknowledgment of their pain and to

be informed about how it can be assessed and managed; and the right of all people with pain to have access to appropriate assessment and treatment of the pain by adequately trained health care professionals. (IASP, 2010)

Another excellent document that practitioners should be aware of that addresses the ethical obligations of health professionals with regards to pain assessment and management is the ethics charter of the American Academy of Pain Medicine (AAPM, 2008).

Medical futility and ethical decision-making

The issue of medical futility is also wrought with controversy in the ethical arena of pain and DOC. One of the issues germane to that discussion, although there are many others, is resource allocation. How much do we allow third-party commercial payers or the legal system or, for that matter, the hospital we work in, to direct or effect decisions regarding whether a patient receives treatment for pain and suffering?

When decisions are made to withdraw or withhold care from someone who is in a state of disordered consciousness, what are the ethical implications with regards to the pain and suffering that the individual may potentially be experiencing (Racine, et al., 2010)? In the context of end-of-life decisions, there remains little controversy regarding pain palliation. From a cultural, religious, political, and medical point of view, there are few who would argue with trying to palliate any significant pain experienced by a person who is dying (i.e., as opposed to being in a static, chronic state of disordered consciousness). There does remain substantive debate about whether conscious awareness in and of itself, including the ability to experience pain and suffering, should be an absolute contraindication for withdrawing or withholding care. In some countries, non-consensual withdrawal of nutrition and hydration in persons with DOC is standard practice, and yet in other countries, such as the US, this phenomenon would create a hailstorm of backlash. Rady and Verheijde (2014) have noted that there is a lack of high-quality research supporting the utility of assisted nutrition and hydration, as well as a lack of knowledge regarding the pain and suffering implications of starvation and dehydration that occur in the context of withdrawing or withholding care and regarding how best to prophylax against the potential for pain and suffering (for more information, see Chapter 7).

Sociocultural and family issues: the ethical challenges

Family conflict is probably one of the most common areas of ethical challenge in the context of managing patients with DOC who are believed to be in pain and/or suffering. How do we balance science and/or consensus regarding these issues with family desires that may be in conflict with physician recommendations? Every clinician will deal with families in which there are conflicting moral, cultural, or religious beliefs about how a given patient with DOC should be treated relative to pain and suffering. The "Holy Grail" of this ethical quagmire is the discussion regarding withholding or withdrawing care directed at pain modulation/alleviation in the context of medical futility. Issues of surrogate consent are also important to acknowledge

Ethics of investigational techniques in assessment and treatment

The debate continues over the limits of information gathered via technology relative to that garnered through bedside physical examination – as related to assessment and clinical decision-making in persons with DOC in general (Fins, 2011) and also more specifically with regards to pain and suffering in this patient population. There remains debate at several levels regarding how much we should and can rely on investigational techniques to assess or treat pain and suffering in persons with DOC. Clinicians must appreciate the ethical tenants associated with the use of investigational techniques and discuss with patient surrogates the risks and benefits, limitations of the science/technology, and surrogates' expectancies (Jox, et al., 2012).

Ethics of research in DOC pain

Biomedical research involving patients with DOC and pain entails a number of ethical as well as legal dimensions that should be considered by all involved in such endeavors (Farisco, et al., 2014). Some have proposed ethical research agenda recommendations as related to persons with DOC in such areas as neuroimaging (Fins, et al., 2008), yet no such recommendations or guidelines for pain research in persons with DOC have yet emerged. A more recent commentary by Farisco et al. (2014) noted a need to look more critically at informed consent procedures, including those for videotaping of persons in DOC who are unable to communicate their own consent.

Ethics in the context of clinicolegal opinions on pain and suffering

Recent advances in neuroimaging and pain assessment clearly have the potential to influence opinions in the context of medicolegal testimony (Luce, 2013). One of the most salient areas of questioning that experts are confronted with in the context of severe brain injury cases is whether a given patient/examinee perceives/feels pain and/or suffers due to that pain. These are difficult questions to answer in a clinical context; however, in a legal context the standard of testimony typically requires that the expert opine with a degree of medical probability, indicating that a given opinion is simply more likely than not. That being said, it is unethical for a clinician to testify to such matters if they have not directly assessed the person in question, ideally serially, and also, optimally, engaged family and significant others in the assessment (Zasler, 2005). It is also of paramount importance that the expert review all relevant neurodiagnostics and relevant records. If there are neurodiagnostics that have not been done that may assist the expert in opining on the issue at hand, then the expert has a professional ethical obligation to inform the triers of this fact. In the context of testimony on pain and suffering in noncommunicative patients in DOC, the limitations of current science must also be adequately acknowledged to the triers of fact (i.e., judge and jury).

Conclusion and directions for the future

The suggested pain perception capacity highlighted by neuroimaging studies in patients in a MCS and in some patients in a VS/UWS supports the idea that these patients need to have their pain generators addressed. Specifically, they need to receive analgesic treatment and/or appropriate pain modulating interventions (whether pharmacological or non-pharmacological), as well as ongoing monitoring. The NCS-R currently represents a rapid, standardized, and sensitive way to behaviorally assess pain in patients with DOC. Complementary pain assessments should nevertheless be developed in order to offer more options to clinicians (see also Chapter 4). While such tools will certainly allow clinicians to prevent and treat pain in this challenging population, they will also lead to developing guidelines that are currently nonexistent and hence crucially needed.

There is still much to be learned and debated regarding the myriad of ethical challenges and conundrums that we face as clinicians treating patients with DOC. The issues of pain and suffering are often some of the most controversial topics in medicine and continue to generate polar opinions, on ethical and other fronts. Further discussion, debate, and research are needed to better equip us to create a rational and ethical set of responses to the various challenges that face us as we collectively address these issues in persons with DOC.

Notes

1 **Nathan D. Zasler,** MD, FAAPM & R, FAADEP, DAAPM, CBIST, is CEO & Medical Director, Concussion Care Centre of Virginia, Ltd.; CEO & Medical Director, Tree of Life Services, Inc.; Professor, affiliate, VCU Department of Physical Medicine and Rehabilitation, Richmond, Virginia; Associate Professor, adjunct, Department of Physical Medicine and Rehabilitation, University of Virginia, Charlottesville, Virginia; Distinguished Clinical Professor of Health Sciences, School of Health Sciences, Touro College, NY; and Vice-Chairperson, IBIA.
2 **Anne T. O'Brien,** Brain Injury Program, Spaulding Rehabilitation Hospital, Boston, MA.
3 **Caroline Schnakers,** PhD, Department of Neurosurgery, University of California–Los Angeles, Los Angeles, CA, USA.

References

American Academy of Pain Medicine. (2008). *Ethics Charter.* Chicago, IL. AAPM.
American Geriatrics Society. (2002). The management of persistent pain in older persons. Clinical practice guideline. *Journal of the American Geriatrics Society*; 50: S205–S224.
Banja JD, Fins JJ. Ethics in brain injury medicine. (2013). In: Zasler ND, Katz DI, Zafonte R (Eds.). *Brain Injury Medicine: Principles and Practice.* Second edition. New York. Demos Publishers. Pp. 1374–1390.

Bernat JL. (2009). Ethical issues in the treatment of severe brain injury: The impact of new technologies. In: Schiff ND, Laureys S (Eds.). *Disorders of Consciousness.* Annals of the New York Academy of Sciences, volume 1157. Boston. Blackwell Publishing. Pp. 117–130.

Bingel U, Quante M, Knab R, et al. (2002). Subcortical structures involved in pain processing: evidence from single-trial fMRI. *Pain;* 99(1–2): 313–321.

Bodart O, Laureys S, Gosseries O. (2013). Coma and disorders of consciousness: scientific advances and practical considerations for clinicians. *Seminars in Neurology;* 33: 83–90.

Boly M, Faymonville ME, Peigneux P, et al. (2005). Cerebral processing of auditory and noxious stimuli in severely brain injured patients: Differences between VS and MCS. In: Coleman MR (Ed.). *The Assessment and Rehabilitation of Vegetative and Minimally Conscious Patients.* New York. Psychology Press. Pp. 283–289.

Boly M, Faymonville ME, Schnakers C, et al. (2008). Perception of pain in the minimally conscious state with PET activation: an observational study. *Lancet Neurology;* 7(11): 1013–1020.

Boly M, Garrido MI, Gosseries O, et al. (2011). Preserved feedforward but impaired top-down processes in the vegetative state. *Science;* 332(6031): 858–862.

Buttner W, Finke W. (2000). Analysis of behavioural and physiological parameters for the assessment of postoperative analgesic demand in newborns, infants and young children: a comprehensive report on seven consecutive studies. *Paediatric Anaesthesia;* 10(3): 303–318.

Chatelle C, Majerus S, Whyte J, et al. (2012). A sensitive scale to assess nociceptive pain in patients with disorders of consciousness. *J Neurol Neurosurg Psychiatry;* 83(12): 1233–1237.

Chatelle C, Thibaut A, Bruno MA, et al. (2014). Nociception Coma Scale-Revised scores correlate with metabolism in the anterior cingulate cortex. *Neurorehabil Neural Repair;* 28(2): 149–152.

Chatelle C, Thibaut A, Whyte J, et al. (2014). Pain issues in disorders of consciousness. *Brain Injury;* 28(9): 1202–1208.

Cruse D, Chennu S, Chatelle C, et al. (2011). Bedside detection of awareness in the vegetative state. *Lancet;* 378(9809): 2088–2094.

Demertzi A, Schnakers C, Ledoux D, et al. (2009). Different beliefs about pain perception in the vegetative and minimally conscious states: a European survey of medical and paramedical professionals. *Progress in Brain Research;* 177: 329–338.

Demertzi A, Laureys S, Bruno MA. (2011). Ethics in disorders of consciousness. In: Vincent JL (Ed.). *Annual Update in Intensive Care and Emergency Medicine.* Berlin. Springer. Pp. 675–682.

Demertzi A, Jox RJ, Racine E, Laureys S. (2014). A European survey on attitudes towards pain and end-of-life issues in locked-in syndrome. *Brain Injury;* 28(9): 1209–1215.

de Tommaso M, Navarro J, Ricci K, et al. (2013). Pain in prolonged disorders of consciousness: laser evoked potentials findings in patients with vegetative and minimally conscious states. *Brain Injury;* 27(7–8): 962–972.

Farisco M, Evers K, Petrini C. (2014). Biomedical research involving patients with disorders of consciousness: ethical and legal dimensions. *Annali dell'Istituto Superiore Di Sanità;* 50(3): 221–228.

Farisco M, Petrini C. (2014). Misdiagnosis as an ethical and scientific challenge. *Annali dell'Istituto Superiore Di Sanità;* 50(3): 229–233.

Fins JJ, Illes J, Bernat JL, et al. (2008). Neuroimaging and disorders of consciousness: envisioning an ethical research agenda. *The American Journal of Bioethics;* 8(9): 3–12.

Fins JJ. (2011). Neuroethics, neuroimaging, and disorders of consciousness: promise or peril? *Transactions of the American Clinical and Climatological Association;* 122: 336–346.

Friedrich O. (2013). Knowledge of partial awareness in disorders of consciousness: implications for ethical evaluations? *Neuroethics*; 6(1): 13–23.

Gelinas C, Johnston C. (2007). Pain assessment in the critically ill ventilated adult: validation of the Critical-Care Pain Observation Tool and physiologic indicators. *Clin J Pain*; 23(6): 497–505.

Gelinas C, Arbour C. (2009). Behavioral and physiologic indicators during a nociceptive procedure in conscious and unconscious mechanically ventilated adults: similar or different? *J Crit Care*; 24(4): 628 e7–17.

Giacino JT, Ashwal S, Childs N, et al. (2002). The minimally conscious state: definition and diagnostic criteria. *Neurology*; 59: 349–353.

Giacino JT, Kalmar K, Whyte J. (2004). The JFK Coma Recovery Scale-Revised: measurement characteristics and diagnostic utility. *Arch Phys Med Rehabil*; 85(12): 2020–2029.

Giacino JT, Katz DI, Whyte J. (2013). Neurorehabilitation in disorders of consciousness. *Seminars in Neurology*; 33(2): 142–156.

Hall JK, Boswell MV. (2009). Ethics, law, and pain management as a patient right. *Pain Physician*; 122(3): 499–506.

Herr KA, Garand L. (2001). Assessment and measurement of pain in older adults. *Clin Geriatr Med*; 17(3): 457–478.

Herr K, Coyne PJ, McCaffery M, et al. (2011). Pain assessment in the patient unable to self-report: position statement with clinical practice recommendations. *Pain Manag Nurs*; 12(4): 230–250.

Hummel P, van Dijk M. (2006). Pain assessment: current status and challenges. *Seminars in Fetal & Neonatal Medicine*; 11: 237–245.

IASP. (1994). *Classification of Chronic Pain: Descriptions of Chronic Pain Syndromes and Definitions of Pain Terms*. Second edition. Seattle. IASP Press.

IASP. (2010). Declaration that access to pain management is a fundamental human right. *J Pain Palliat Care Pharmacother*; 25(1): 29–31.

Institute of Medicine. (2011). *Relieving Pain in America: A Blueprint for Transforming Prevention, Care, Education and Research*. Washington, DC. The National Academies Press.

Jennett B, Plum F. (1972). Persistent vegetative state after brain damage: a syndrome in search of a name. *Lancet*; 1: 734–737.

Jox RJ, Bernat JL, Laureys S, Racine E. (2012). Disorders of consciousness: responding to requests for novel diagnostic and therapeutic interventions. *Lancet Neurology*; 11(8): 732–738.

Kassubek J, Juengling FD, Els T, et al. (2003). Activation of a residual cortical network during painful stimulation in long-term postanoxic vegetative state: a ^{15}O–H$_2$O PET study. *J Neurol Sci*; 212(1–2): 85–91.

Kotchoubey B, Merz S, Lang S, et al. (2013). Global functional connectivity reveals highly significant differences between the vegetative and the minimally conscious state. *J Neurol*; 260(4): 975–983.

Lanzillo B, Loreto V, Calabrese C, et al. (2014). Does pain relief influence recovery of consciousness? A case report of a patient's treatment with ziconotide. *Eur J Phys Rehabil Med*; Epub ahead of print.

Laureys S, Faymonville ME, Luxen A, et al. (2000). Restoration of thalamocortical connectivity after recovery from persistent vegetative state. *Lancet*; 355: 1790–1791.

Laureys S, Faymonville M, Peigneux P, et al. (2002). Cortical processing of noxious somatosensory stimuli in the persistent vegetative state. *Neuroimage*; 17(2): 732–741.

Laureys S, Tononi G (Eds.). (2009). *The Neurology of Consciousness: Cognitive Neuroscience and Neuropathology*. Boston. Elsevier.

Loeser JD, Treede RD. (2008). The Kyoto protocol of IASP basic pain terminology. *Pain*; 137(3): 473–477.

Luce JM. (2013). Chronic disorders of consciousness following coma: part two: ethical, legal, and social issues. *Chest*; 144(4): 1388–1393.

Lutkenhoff ES, McArthur DL, Hua X, et al. (2013). Thalamic atrophy in antero-medial and dorsal nuclei correlates with six-month outcome after severe brain injury. *Neuroimage Clin*; 3: 396–404.

Markl A, Yu T, Vogel D, et al. (2013). Brain processing of pain in patients with unresponsive wakefulness syndrome. *Brain Behav*; 3(2): 95–103.

Monti MM, Vanhaudenhuyse A, Coleman MR, et al. (2010). Willful modulation of brain activity in disorders of consciousness. *N Engl J Med*; 362(7): 579–589.

Nakase-Richardson R, Whyte J, Giacino JT, et al. (2012). Longitudinal outcome of patients with disordered consciousness in the NIDRR TBI Model Systems Programs. *Journal of Neurotrauma*; 29(1): 59–65.

Pew Research Religion & Public Life Project. (2013). Religious groups' views on end-of-life issues. http://www.pewforum.org/2013/11/21/religious-groups-views-on-end-of-life-issues/

Pistoia F, Sacco S, Sara M, Carolei A. (2013). The perception of pain and its management in disorders of consciousness. *Curr Pain Headache Rep*; 17(374): 1–10.

Pistoia F, Sacco S, Sara M, et al. (2015). Intrathecal baclofen: Effects on spasticity, pain, and consciousness in disorders of consciousness and locked-in syndrome. *Curr Pain Headache Rep*; 19(1): 466.

Posner JB, Saper CD, Schiff ND, Plum F. (2007). *Plum and Posner's Diagnosis of Stupor and Coma*. Fourth edition. *Contemporary Neurology Series*. New York. Oxford University Press.

Racine E, Rodrigue C, Bernat JL, et al. (2010). Observations on the ethical and social aspects of disorders of consciousness. *The Canadian Journal of Neurological Sciences*; 37(6): 758–768.

Racine E. (2013). Pragmatic neuroethics: the social aspects of ethics in disorders of consciousness. *Handbook of Clinical Neurology*; 118: 357–372.

Rady MY, Verheijde JL. (2014). Non-consensual withdrawal of nutrition and hydration in prolonged disorders of consciousness: authoritarianism and trustworthiness in medicine. *Philosophy, Ethics, and Humanities in Medicine*; 9(1): 16.

Sattin D, Pagani M, Covelli V, et al. (2013). The Italian version of the Nociception Coma Scale. *Int J Rehabil Res*; 36(2): 182–186.

Shackman AJ, Salomons TV, Slagter HA, et al. (2011). The integration of negative affect, pain and cognitive control in the cingulate cortex. *Nat Rev Neurosci*; 12(3): 154–167.

Schnakers C, Zasler ND. (2007). Pain assessment and management in disorders of consciousness. *Current Opinion in Neurology*; 20(6): 620–626.

Schnakers C, Perrin F, Schabus M, et al. (2009). Detecting consciousness in a total locked-in syndrome: an active event-related paradigm. *Neurocase*; 15(4): 271–277.

Schnakers C, Vanhaudenhuyse A, Giacino J, et al. (2009). Diagnostic accuracy of the vegetative and minimally conscious state: clinical consensus versus standardized neurobehavioral assessment. *BMC Neurol*; 9: 35.

Schnakers C, Chatelle C, Vanhaudenhuyse A, et al. (2010). The Nociception Coma Scale: a new tool to assess nociception in disorders of consciousness. *Pain*; 148(2): 215–219.

Shewmon DA. (2004). A critical analysis of conceptual domains of the vegetative state: sorting fact from fancy. *NeuroRehabilitation*; 19(4): 335–348.

The Multi-Society Task Force on PVS. (1994). Medical aspects of the persistent vegetative state (1). *N Engl J Med*; 330(21): 1499–1508.

Thibaut A, Chatelle C, Wannez S, et al. (2014). Spasticity in disorders of consciousness: a behavioral study. *Eur J Phys Rehabil Med*; Epub ahead of print.

Vink P, Eskes AM, Lindeboom R, et al. (2014). Nurses assessing pain with the Nociception Coma Scale: interrater reliability and validity. *Pain Manag Nurs*; 15(4): 881–887.

Warden V, Hurley AC, Volicer L. (2003). Development and psychometric evaluation of the Pain Assessment In Advanced Dementia (PAINAD) Scale. *Journal of the American Medical Directors Association*; 4(1): 9–15.

Young J, Siffleet J, Nikoletti S, Shaw T. (2006). Use of a Behavioural Pain Scale to assess pain in ventilated, unconscious and/or sedated patients. *Intensive Crit Care Nurs*; 22(1): 32–39.

Yu T, Lang S, Vogel D, et al. (2013). Patients with unresponsive wakefulness syndrome respond to the pain cries of other people. *Neurology*; 80(4): 345–352.

Zasler, ND. (2005). Forensic assessment issues in low level neurological states. *Neuropsychological Rehabilitation*; 15(3/4): 251–256.

Zasler ND, Martelli MF, Nicholson K. (2013). Post-traumatic pain disorders: Medical assessment and management. In: Zasler ND, Katz DI, Zafonte R (Eds.). *Brain Injury Medicine: Principles and Practice*. Second edition. New York. Demos Publishers. Pp. 954–973.

4 Overcoming the challenges of accurately assessing consciousness and communication in the context of pain assessment

John Whyte[1] *and Mark Sherer*[2]

Abbreviations

CRS-R   Coma Recovery Scale-Revised
DOC   disorders of consciousness
MCS   minimally conscious state
PTCS   post-traumatic confusional state
QIBA   Quantitative Individualized Behavioral Assessment
TBI   traumatic brain injury
VS   vegetative state

Introduction

Severe brain injury typically leads to unconsciousness (coma). Coma may be relatively brief and evolve directly into higher states of consciousness over a period of days. In the most severe cases, coma may evolve into the vegetative state and only later, if at all, transition into the minimally conscious state (MCS), the confusional state, and higher states of consciousness (Whyte, Ponsford, Watanabe, & Hart, 2010). In disorders of consciousness (DOC), the pace of recovery is highly variable, and some patients may spend prolonged intervals in a given state of consciousness or even plateau there indefinitely (Giacino & Whyte, 2005). Behavioral and physiologic responses in DOC patients are often quite variable, which makes it difficult to distinguish random fluctuations from more consistent trends in recovery or deterioration.

Patients with severe brain injury may also suffer from coexisting conditions that produce nociceptive stimulation. This is particularly true for patients whose DOC results from traumatic brain injury (TBI), since the same trauma may produce fractures, damage to internal organs, nerve lesions, etc. (Whyte et al., 2010). Though less common after nontraumatic injuries, such patients are still at risk for a range of unrelated painful conditions, such as kidney stones, bowel obstruction, or urinary tract infection, which would normally be heralded by localizing pain responses.

In this context, it is important to carefully characterize the level of consciousness and communication abilities of a patient in DOC, and it is also important to monitor for the presence of noxious stimuli and subjective pain. But level of consciousness affects the processing of noxious stimulation as subjective pain, and this, in turn, highlights the fact that the evaluation of these two issues (consciousness/communication and nociception/pain) is intertwined. Should one attempt to definitively characterize consciousness first in order to know how to interpret possible signs of pain? Or should one attempt to assess the presence of noxious stimuli first, irrespective of the state of consciousness? The answer to these questions, we would argue, depends on the acuity of the brain injury that produces a DOC.

In the early period after injury, nociception is an important indicator of potential medical comorbidities, whether or not the patient subjectively experiences pain. That is, even if a patient were definitely known to be unconscious, one would still want to treat a fracture or remove an inflamed appendix to optimize the chances for further functional recovery. Thus, whether the patient subjectively perceives pain at this point in time is a lower priority issue. In contrast, in a patient whose DOC persists for many months it may be ethically and legally important to assess the capacity for subjective pain and suffering and not merely the presence of physiologic nociception. Moreover, in the early period post-injury, it is likely that a DOC may evolve fairly rapidly. Thus, even if a painstaking assessment of consciousness is done, the result of that assessment may soon become obsolete. It is unwise to conclude that a patient is incapable of subjective pain on an ongoing basis based on an assessment at a point in time.

The evaluation of a patient in DOC, then, should attempt to answer three questions:

1 What is the patient's current level of consciousness and communication and pace of evolution?
2 What evidence exists for the presence of nociceptive stimuli?
3 How does the current level of consciousness and communication affect the interpretation of behavioral evidence of nociception?

Challenges in assessing consciousness

Consciousness cannot be directly observed. It must be inferred from the relationship between patterns of events in the environment and patterns of behavior in the patient. That is, when we say, for shorthand, that "the patient follows commands," we can't actually observe any direct linkage between the instructions of the examiner and the movements of the patient. Rather, we note the fact that a movement corresponding to the examiner's request occurred soon after and we infer that the instruction "caused" the movement. In reality, this assumption relies on the *contingent relationship* between the environmental event (the utterance of the examiner's instructions) and the patient's behavior (the occurrence of the requested movement) (Giacino et al., 2002). This contingent relationship is a statistical concept meaning that the probability of observing a particular patient movement in the presence of the relevant command is higher than the probability of observing it with no such command present. With higher-level patients, this statistical "computation" is implicit. If a cooperative patient claps her hands three times upon request, we already know that as we walk around the hospital ward we are unlikely to see patients clapping their hands three times without such a command. But if the command is "blink your eyes" and we see an eye blink, we are much less confident because of the awareness that eye blinks in the absence of such a command are very common. Since many patients with DOC are only capable of very simple behaviors such as eye blinks or limb movements, we may need to rely on actual statistical comparisons rather than assumed statistical differences to determine whether such a contingent relationship exists.

Each time we indicate to a patient (whether verbally, by demonstration, etc.) that we want them to perform some behavior, we are implicitly testing an entire "input-output chain." That is, for a patient to follow our request requires them to process the visual or verbal instruction, to compute the correct response, and to plan and execute the requested motor response. Thus, successful performance establishes the integrity (at least at that level of difficulty) of the entire chain. Failure to emit the desired behavior, in contrast, tells us that the chain is broken but not which step is responsible for the break. The patient could have failed to hear the instruction, attend to it, understand its meaning, plan the motor response, or launch the actual movement, to name just the gross steps involved. As a corollary, then, we can gather definitive evidence supporting the presence of consciousness, but we can never gather definitive evidence proving the absence of consciousness. We can only repeatedly fail to establish its presence, but the search for consciousness is never, strictly speaking, "complete." Because of this, when we fail in our attempts to document the presence of consciousness, it is important to consider the other confounding impairments (e.g., deafness, aphasia, apraxia) that might have interfered with the detection of consciousness.

Challenges in assessing communication

In routine clinical practice, assessment of pain generally involves communication between the patient and health-care provider. The patient is asked to provide a history of the pain, including such factors as when it started, what provoked it, what makes it better and worse, etc. (Smith et al., 2015). They are also asked to localize the pain to a body part and to characterize the nature of the pain (e.g., "stabbing," "crushing," "aching," etc.). Finally, patients are typically asked to rate the severity of their pain on a visual analog pain scale, which helps the practitioner track its fluctuations and assess its relationship to maneuvers intended to treat or modify the pain. However, these various forms of communication can all be affected by severe brain injury. Patients may fail to communicate important clues about the nature and severity of their pain. But their cognitive and communication problems may also lead them to over report pain. Thus, it is important to carefully characterize the patient's cognitive and communication abilities as they relate to the ability to report on subjective pain, and to consider alternative sources of evidence about pain where these abilities are found to be unreliable.

A number of general and specific impairments can compromise ability to communicate in persons recovering from severe brain injury. General impairments include inadequate awareness of self and environment, inadequate level of arousal, and diffuse impairment of attention. More specific impairments include primary sensory deficits such as severely impaired hearing and/or vision; motor impairments such as dysarthria, motor weakness, spasticity, and/or lack of head and neck control; primary language impairment (i.e., aphasia); and disorders of initiation (e.g., akinetic mutism). As with other functional abilities, the ability to communicate may be quite fragile in early recovery so that factors such as fatigue, excessive stimulation, physical condition (e.g., constipation, urinary tract infection, etc.), and others can cause fluctuation in communication from day to day, at different times in the same day, or even minute to minute in the same assessment session. A number of factors that affect communication can co-occur in persons with diffuse brain injury caused by anoxia or trauma. Those with large lesions due to hemispheric stroke may also have complex impairments of communication abilities. This co-occurrence of various impairments complicates the development of strategies to maximize communicative abilities in the severely impaired patient.

Ability to communicate is not sufficient to permit assessment of pain. Pain assessment may begin with whether or not the patient is experiencing pain in the moment, but the overall assessment is more complex. Whether or not the patient is currently experiencing pain, the health-care provider will want to know if the patient has sustained pain in the recent past, the location and nature of the pain, how the recent pain compares to pain experienced in the past, factors that worsen or lessen the pain, the extent to which pain limits ability to participate in functional activities, and other details. Even when communication abilities are relatively intact, impaired memory, excessive emotionality, distractibility, and other factors can make accurate assessment of pain and response to pain therapies difficult.

Sensitive methods for assessing consciousness

There are two broad approaches to the behavioral assessment of consciousness: standardized assessment and individualized assessment. Each has advantages and disadvantages, and the ideal assessment repertoire probably includes elements of both approaches. Standardized and individualized assessment will both be discussed below, but first we address some issues of clinical context that are equally pertinent to both assessment approaches.

General health context

A wide variety of medical conditions may affect alertness and consciousness. Many clinicians report that relatively common conditions, such as a urinary tract infection or pneumonia, may lead to behavioral regression in patients hovering at the boundary between VS/UWS and MCS. Technically speaking, an assessment that finds a medically ill patient to be unconscious is not "inaccurate," but that level of consciousness may underestimate the patient's neurologic capacity. Thus, the first line of care for patients with early DOC is to optimize their overall level of health, while choosing treatments that minimize adverse central nervous system side effects.

Confounding impairments

As noted above, behavioral assessment of consciousness is an asymmetrical affair: empirical evidence can support the presence of consciousness but cannot prove its absence. Moreover, failure at a given assessment task doesn't specify which link in the input-output chain is broken. Thus, the approach to behavioral assessment should consider other processing impairments that may be present by virtue of the location of focal central nervous system lesions or by virtue of premorbid or comorbid injuries or conditions.

Beginning with a complete medical history, one should assess the presence of premorbid sensory, motor, or cognitive impairments. Older patients, especially, may have significant hearing impairments that could interfere with language comprehension. Patients of any age may have difficulty looking at or responding to visual stimuli if they are not wearing glasses (and glasses are particularly likely to be lost in traumatic injuries). Premorbid neurologic conditions such as poliomyelitis or Parkinson's Disease may interfere with the ability to execute certain motor commands. And of course pre-injury intellectual impairment may limit the level of functioning that might be expected.

The history of the injury or illness that resulted in the DOC is equally relevant. As mentioned above, patients with traumatic DOC may have impairments caused by other forms of co-occurring trauma. They may be visually impaired because of orbital fractures and optic nerve trauma. They may suffer brachial plexus injury or other peripheral nerve injury that interferes with motor execution. Co-occurring spinal cord injury may limit behavioral response more profoundly. Moreover, the history of illness or injury may suggest possible sources of pain related to fractures, nerve lesions, or internal injuries.

In the case of both traumatic and nontraumatic DOC, one must also consider what brain lesions might produce confounding impairments. Large left peri-sylvian lesions may limit comprehension of spoken language and, thus, the ability to respond to verbal commands (National Institutes of Health, 2008). Left hemisphere lesions may also produce apraxia that may interfere with the patient's ability to form a motor response (Barrett & Foundas, 2004). Right parietal lesions may make it difficult for the patient to attend to and respond to left-sided stimuli (Buxbaum et al., 2004). Deep hemispheric lesions or occipital pole lesions may produce field cuts or cortical blindness, rendering the patient unresponsive to visual stimuli (Celesia & Brigell, 2005). Bi-frontal lesions may severely undermine initiation of responses to many stimuli (Nagaratnam, Nagaratnam, Ng, & Diu, 2004). In addition, patients with prolonged stays in the intensive care unit due to any cause are at risk for critical illness neuropathy, which may limit motor responses (Latronico & Bolton, 2011).

Carefully considering the patient's premorbid functioning, as well as the possible presence of these confounding deficits, allows the clinician to design an assessment that "works around" or controls for some of these confounds, or at least alerts one to the need to consider other sources of difficulty in responding.

As noted, this consideration begins with a thorough review of the premorbid and current history. Neuroimaging studies are an essential source of information about brain lesions that may be associated with other confounding impairments. For this purpose, it is helpful to review not only the acute imaging studies, but also to review imaging of the residual neuropathology after acute medical or surgical treatment. Electrophysiologic measures (e.g., visual evoked responses, electromyography for critical illness neuropathy) may help to establish injury to specific sensory or motor pathways in selected cases.

Physical examination provides a great deal of guidance, particularly about the patient's motor function. Simple observation of the patient without interaction can be extremely informative. A patient's limbs may be in decorticate or decerebrate postures, and this positioning is a rough guide to the types of motor responses that might be expected from such patients even if conscious. Flaccid or atrophic limbs may suggest peripheral nerve injury or critical illness neuropathy. On the other hand, a patient may be seen to finger bed sheets or medical tubes in ways that suggest a rudimentary "purpose" and adaptability to the environment, and that could support more sophisticated motor responses such as pointing. Head posture and degree of lid opening suggest the patient's level of arousal, though specific neck muscle or lid muscle paralysis may give an incorrect impression. Patients who are frequently under aroused, in particular, should have their medications reviewed for agents with potentially sedating effects.

The position and movement of the eyes may also be informative. If the eyes are tonically deviated far to one side, the use of eye movements to signal consciousness may be unwise, and the deviation may suggest a more fundamental difficulty with processing visual information. The range of eye movements seen spontaneously or in response to head movements provides a guide to the patient's underlying capacities for eye movement (e.g., could the patient be asked to look up/down or left/right?). The spontaneous frequency and magnitude of all of the patient's movements are important to evaluate. Movements that are spontaneously very common will be difficult to evaluate as responses to command requests. On the other hand, movements that have never been seen may be beyond the patient's movement capacity irrespective of level of consciousness. Movements that are very small in magnitude may pose problems for clinical agreement about whether or not a response occurred. Thus, the ideal movements to explore as voluntary signals of consciousness are easily discernible movements that occur with low to moderate frequency.

Finally, family members and professional caregivers should be interviewed to identify any observations that may suggest evidence of consciousness. Often, these reports will include multiple behaviors that may be erroneously attributed to consciousness (e.g., the patient opens her eyes when stimulated, the patient yawns, the patient grimaces during suctioning, the patient blinks on command, etc.). However, careful questioning may sharpen these observational reports. For example, if a patient's mouth opens or moves when touched with a spoon, this may be a reflexive response. But if the patient's mouth opens as a spoon approaches, this suggests some level of visual recognition of the spoon and awareness of its function. In most instances, observations by family members and nonexpert clinicians will need to be carefully verified, but at the very least they inform hypotheses about where the evidence of consciousness might be found.

Physical examination provides information not only about probable state of consciousness and factors that may interfere with its accurate assessment, but also about possible sources of pain. For example, physical examination may reveal swelling or redness in a limb suggestive of fracture or heterotopic ossification, the presence of pressure sores, or the presence of incisions indicative of recent invasive procedures.

Upon completion of this preliminary evaluation, the examiner will be able to synthesize a list of behaviors that may lie within the patient's repertoire if the patient is conscious, as well as a list of behaviors that may be difficult for the patient to produce irrespective of level of consciousness, and this allows a systematic behavioral assessment to be planned while optimally avoiding the pitfalls of confounding deficits. On the one hand, when one wishes to optimize the chance of detecting consciousness, one might attempt to provide multiple sources of information to compensate for possible limitations in processing specific sources. For example, one might deliver verbal commands along with gestures since a response to either one suggests consciousness. On the other hand, one might seek to document that there is a specific confounding impairment. In that case, one could assess command-following to purely verbal stimuli as compared to the combination of verbal and gestural stimuli and interpret a difference in accuracy as evidence of a coexisting aphasia.

Standardized assessment of consciousness

Over the last two decades, a number of specialized assessments of consciousness have been developed specifically to improve the objectivity and reliability of the assessment of patients with DOC. Available assessment tools vary in many ways, including administration time, level of training needed, and functional level targeted (Seel et al., 2010). Importantly, these tools differ in terms of whether they dictate specific examiner behaviors and specific patient responses required for scoring, or whether they simply ask the examiner to rate the patient's behavior using their own clinical judgment. For example, the Coma Recovery

Scale-Revised (CRS-R) requires that one issue specific commands to look at or reach for a named object or to move a specific body part and requires that the patient perform the requested behavior a specific number of times to be scored (Giacino, Kalmar, & Whyte, 2004). At the other extreme, the Disability Rating Scale item for command-following suggests finger movement as the test behavior but allows for the selection of any other behavior if that isn't suitable and provides no guidance about how many times the patient must display the required behavior (Rappaport, Hall, Hopkins, Belleza, & Cope, 1982). Rather, scoring of this scale is based on the examiner's judgment that any behaviors that were observed were in response to the command given.

As a general principle, we favor scales that operationally define the examiner's behavior and the patient's required responses, since this reduces the chance for subjective bias in scoring as well as the possibility of increased score variability caused by selection of commands or behaviors that differ in difficulty. In an evidence-based review of existing assessment scales for patients with DOC several scales met this overall condition, but the CRS-R received the highest rating based on the available evidence.

Standardized scales have a number of advantages. Because of their standard administration structure, it is possible to train frontline staff to conduct these assessments and for them to acquire a volume of experience from repeatedly administering the same scale to multiple patients. Also, standardized scales tend to survey a broad range of behavioral domains so they are likely to detect improvement or deterioration in whatever domain is changing. In addition, using a standardized scale on all patients facilitates program evaluation and observational research, since the same data elements are available on all of the patients in a program.

In Figure 4.1, below, we show data from regular administration of the CRS-R. The patient is a 28-year-old male pedestrian who was struck by a car. Glasgow Coma Score in the emergency department was three. Blood was noted in the left ear canal, indicating a basilar skull fracture. A CT scan revealed evidence of diffuse axonal injury with small scattered intraparenchymal hematomas, as well as bilateral orbital fractures. Intracranial pressure was difficult to control and he was ultimately treated with a bi-frontal craniectomy. He was admitted to an acute inpatient rehabilitation facility 40 days post-injury. At the time of admission there was still pronounced swelling of the brain, causing bulging of the scalp over the craniectomy site. His initial CRS-R score was four, consistent with the VS, but over the ensuing weeks, despite the swelling, he showed clear and relatively consistent functional improvement. He suffered a generalized seizure 37 days after admission. A follow-up CT scan showed ventricular enlargement, and although it was difficult to determine whether this reflected brain atrophy or hydrocephalus, he was started on levetiracetam and received a ventriculoperitoneal shunt. Over the next few weeks, the craniectomy site became increasingly concave. Despite the seizure, shunt, and sunken scalp flap, his functional improvement continued. However, 82 days after admission he suffered two more generalized seizures and was transferred to acute care for management. A head CT on this occasion revealed asymmetrical enlargement

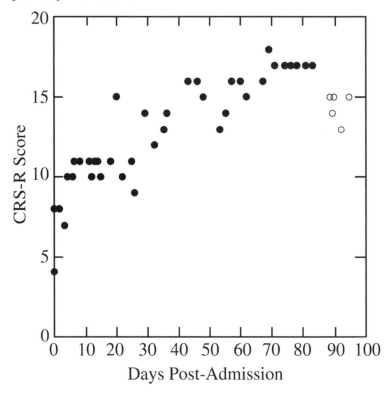

Figure 4.1 Total score on the Coma Recovery Scale-Revised (CRS-R) is shown on the Y-axis and the days post-admission to rehabilitation on the X-axis. The filled circles show a clear trend toward improved functioning, after which a decline is shown with unfilled circles.

of the left lateral ventricle and early protrusion of left-brain tissue into the craniectomy site. He was started on lacosamide and he returned to the rehabilitation facility while awaiting scheduling of a cranioplasty and shunt revision in the hopes that this would help manage fluctuations in intracranial pressure. CRS-R scores during this interval were consistently several points lower than prior to the seizure, suggesting impairment of consciousness caused by some combination of brain hemodynamic changes, postictal effects, and/or the effects of the second anticonvulsant. These data illustrate the sensitivity of the trajectory of quantitative measures of consciousness, such as the CRS-R, to adverse events. Changes in scores on quantitative measures can prompt a search for medical comorbidities even in the absence of obvious signs such as seizures.

Standardized scales also have some limitations. As noted, the definition of MCS hinges on a contingent relationship between environmental events and patient behavior, but this contingent relationship can be in any content domain. Thus, a patient who smiles and laughs at jokes but not at non-humorous content would meet the definition of MCS, but if this is the only behavior that satisfies the definition of MCS it is unlikely to be detected by a standardized scale. Second, a standardized scale can only go so far in "working around" confounding deficits. For example, in the CRS-R's "auditory function scale" the examiner is provided with three command options: to look at a named object, to reach for a named object, or to move a named body part. The availability of looking at or reaching for options helps work around patients who have limitations in eye movements or limb movements. The option of body part commands helps work around patients who may have visual impairment. But of course the patient who has severe receptive aphasia may not be able to understand any of those commands. Finally, standardized scales typically have relatively few scoring options within a domain. To use the example of the CRS-R auditory function scale again, a patient who responds to three of four commands will get a score of three; a patient who responds to four instances of two different commands promptly will get a score of four. But what about a patient who responds to two of four commands? Or a patient who responds to four instances of one command but only three instances of another? These intermediate levels of performance are not scored and the score does not appear to change until a new criterion is reached.

Individualized assessment of consciousness

The principles of single–subject experimental design, or "N–of–1 research," can also be applied to the assessment of patients with DOC. Essentially this involves formulating hypotheses about what the relationship should be between specific environmental events and specific patient behaviors *if the patient is conscious*, and then testing these hypotheses empirically with individualized data collection under a patient-specific protocol. Over a number of years we have developed an approach, based on this logic, entitled Quantitative Individualized Behavioral Assessment (QIBA). We have applied this approach to the assessment of vision and visual attention, auditory command-following, and even the detection of humor perception, and we provide several case examples of these applications below (Whyte & DiPasquale, 1995; Whyte, DiPasquale, & Vaccaro, 1999; Whyte, Laborde, & DiPasquale, 1999).

    The advantages and disadvantages of QIBA are virtually the mirror image of standardized approaches. Because QIBA is, by definition, individualized, any confounding deficits can be assessed or controlled for as long as the examiner can conceive of an assessment design with the appropriate control conditions. For example, when assessing a patient's awareness of the function of objects, one may have difficulty if the patient has sufficient proximal weakness that she can't raise a brush to the hair or a cup to the lips. One might then consider a set of objects that are all used at table height but in very different ways. For example, one might choose a pen and scissors. Second, one may design assessment protocols to evaluate uncommon behaviors that are not found on standardized scales. We had the opportunity to assess a woman whose family believed that she responded to humorous events but showed no other signs of consciousness beyond intermittent visual pursuit. We collected video clips of comedy shows and video clips of news programs and developed operational criteria for scoring "smiling" and "laughing." When she was randomly shown short segments of the different forms of programming, there was a significantly higher frequency of smiling and laughing in response to humorous videos than to news programs, verifying her conscious perception of humor. Another advantage of QIBA is the ability to detect subtle and continuous change within an assessment domain. For example, if one is assessing command-following in response to a defined set of commands, one can compute the percentage of commands followed each day and have a continuous measure of increasing (or decreasing) reliability of command-following rather than two or three categorical ratings. This is particularly helpful when exploring the relationship between behavioral performance and medical events or psychoactive medications.

Table 4.1 shows data gathered during a command-following protocol. This patient had only one behavior (lifting a thumb) that was thought to possibly be volitional. Thus, we constructed a protocol with three kinds of trials delivered in random order: "Lift your thumb," "Hold still," or [silent observation]. We also defined what constituted a scorable thumb movement and hypothesized that if the movement was under conscious control it should be seen more frequently in the "Lift" condition than either of the other two. The inclusion of a "Hold still" condition controlled for the possibility that noise alone would stimulate more spontaneous movement. Note that while the frequency of movement is low in all conditions, it is significantly more frequent in the expected condition.

Figure 4.2 shows command-following data over time to illustrate that the reliability of command-following changes gradually during recovery. The patient is a 32-year-old man who was injured in a fall of 20–30 feet. He suffered a seizure at the scene. On evaluation at the trauma center, he had a Glasgow Coma Score of five, and a CT scan revealed a right epidural hematoma with right to left shift, as well as multiple contusions. A craniectomy was performed, along with evacuation of the hematoma, but an early cranioplasty was performed six weeks post-injury and he was admitted to rehabilitation 10 weeks post-injury. On admission he was thought to occasionally touch his head or move his leg

Table 4.1 Data collected during a command-following protocol based on the Quantitative Individualized Behavioral Assessment.

Command condition	Lifts thumb	No response	Number of trials
"Lift your thumb"	**49**	**48**	97
"Hold still"	**12**	**83**	95
[Silent observation]	**12**	**84**	96
Total	73	215	288

Chi Square, 2 d.f. = 49, p<.0001

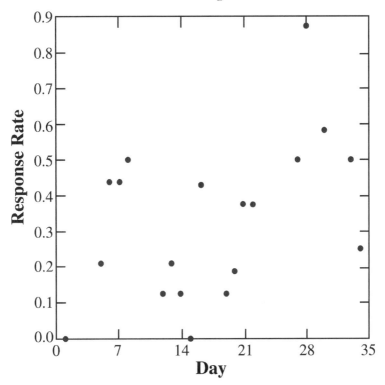

Figure 4.2 The patient's response rate (number of commands followed/number of commands given) is plotted on the Y-axis, and the day of data collection (beginning with the first day of the assessment protocol) on the X-axis. Note the extreme day-to-day variability in responding, despite a general trend toward increased responding over time.

on command. Therefore, a dual-command protocol was begun in which he was randomly requested to "touch your head" or "move your leg." Each trial was scored as "no response," a head touch, or a leg movement. In general it was found that he made few errors but failed to respond at all on a substantial number of trials (see Figure 4.2 for a plot of his response rate [proportion of trials on which he responded]).

QIBA also has some disadvantages. The individualization that is its primary virtue also means that each assessment involves designing a rigorous controlled "experiment." If designing well-controlled experiments were a simple endeavor, we would probably have a much larger volume of evidence by now! To implement QIBA well in a clinical environment, therefore, requires the availability of a staff member with relatively advanced protocol design and statistical analysis skills who can support frontline team members in data collection and make use of their invaluable clinical observations in shaping the design.

Because developing the optimal design for a protocol can be challenging, there is also the tendency for team members to gradually shift their focus from, "What question do we need to answer, and what protocol would help us answer it?" to "What protocols do we have already designed that we could try out on this patient?" with the corresponding risk that the available tools drive the evaluation rather than the clinical needs of the patient. Finally, because QIBA tends to focus the assessments on specific domains or questions of interest, it can only detect change in the domains being tracked. Thus, one might have the experience that the reliability of command-following does not appear to be improving but there are anecdotal reports that the patient is engaging in more functional object use. Since there was no QIBA protocol being run regarding functional object use, one is left with reliance on subjective impressions.

An integrated approach

We have suggested that the optimal assessment approach combines standardized and individualized assessment. Particularly in the case of patients who appear to be in the VS/UWS on admission, it may be difficult to select a domain for QIBA because nothing in particular is a promising or interesting behavior. For VS patients, surely, it is important to conduct a broad functional assessment so that one can be alert to domains where change is occurring. We recommend that all patients with DOC be administered a standardized assessment daily or several times per week when first admitted in order to characterize their current level of functioning, rate of change, and degree of day-to-day variability. Once behaviors appear that are suggestive of consciousness or that are clinically ambiguous or perplexing, QIBA protocols that explore these in more depth can be added, and these will also serve as more sensitive indicators of change within these targeted domains. The frequency of standardized assessment may be reduced to weekly once more is known about specific cognitive and behavioral domains, as the standardized assessment becomes less relevant as a diagnostic tool and more relevant as a global measure of the rate of progress.

The integration of these two approaches will allow the clinician to answer a range of questions, including some of the following, that go beyond the current state of consciousness:

- What is the patient's current DOC diagnosis?
- How much does the patient's level of consciousness fluctuate from day to day or hour to hour?
- Is the patient's level of consciousness changing and at what rate?
- What sensory, motor, and/or cognitive impairments exist in addition to a disorder of consciousness and what are the most effective ways of bypassing or accommodating these additional impairments?
- Does the patient's current level of consciousness (along with coexisting impairments) support some form of reliable communication and, if so, what is the best approach to communication?

- Does the patient's current level of consciousness (along with coexisting impairments) allow for some form of functional engagement with the environment and, if so, what is the optimal approach for achieving functional performance?

Assessing the accuracy of communication

As with assessment of consciousness, initial assessment of the patient's capacity for communication begins by determining whether various conditions that would eliminate or compromise the ability to communicate are present. By definition, persons in the VS do not communicate as they lack awareness of self and the environment and may have a host of conditions that would limit ability to communicate (Giacino et al., 2002). However, even in the VS there may be some findings that could be pertinent to later assessment of communication. Does the patient appear to be hemiparetic? Are the eyes deviated to the right? Does the patient show a startle response to loud sounds? Does the patient show pathologic posturing to aversive stimulation?

Early transition from the VS is usually indicated by visual fixation and pursuit and/or a localization response to noxious stimuli (Van Erp et al., 2015). Presence of fixation and pursuit suggests that the visual system is to some extent intact, and presence of a localization response suggests that there is ability to make discrete movements with at least one limb. Patients who are not intubated may phonate when given noxious stimulation to elicit the localization response. Since speech is always the preferred medium for communication presence of phonation can be an encouraging sign, but presence of the ability to control eye movements and/or the ability to make discrete limb or head movements indicate possible alternative routes for obtaining yes/no responses.

Initial attempts at eliciting communication usually focus on command-following and establishing a consistent yes/no response. One can perform a very simple assessment of hearing by presenting a loud sound such as clapping hands outside the patient's view. If a startle response is shown, the patient has at least some limited ability to hear. However, this response can be mediated at the brainstem level and may not indicate conscious awareness of sound (Yeomans & Frankland, 1996). Once an auditory startle is established, more subtle sounds such as a finger rub can be presented to one side and then the other to determine if the patient will localize to sound. Demonstration of localization to sound suggests that the patient has at least limited conscious awareness of sound or has the potential to develop this awareness.

Accurate command-following provides clear evidence that the patient can process language at, at least, a rudimentary level. Similarly, the ability to give yes/no responses suggests some understanding of language as well as some degree of communicative intent. Once an adequate level of arousal is achieved, most patients will give some indication of an intention to communicate. This could take the form of phonation even if no words can be recognized, pointing, head nods and/or shakes, facial expressions, or other gestures. In our experience, indication of an intention to communicate is a positive sign and is likely to be associated with additional recovery. Patients may fail to demonstrate intention to communicate due to continuing in the VS, to inadequate level of arousal, to aphasia, or to impaired initiation such as that associated with akinetic mutism.

Yes/no responding

Since the most basic pain assessment is "Are you in pain?" early assessment of pain depends on establishing a reliable yes/no response. If the patient shows any evidence at all that he/she can answer yes/no or give distinguishable headshakes and nods, these response modalities should be pursued. Any substituted mode of response requires at least some element of new learning and engagement of motor and sensory mechanisms not normally required for yes/no responding. If the patient cannot give intelligible yes/no responses due to intubation or dysarthria and the patient does not have adequate head control to give headshakes and nods, other modalities can be tried. The most common alternatives are thumbs up for yes, thumbs down for no, and pointing to or fixing the eyes on the words "yes" and "no" when they are presented in a visual field and at an eye level that the patient has shown consistent ability to respond to. Other alternatives, such as eye blinks and leg movements, do not have the virtue of being overlearned behaviors and depend on some learning and conscious mediation.

Regardless of modality, initial trials of yes/no responding should begin with questions about the patient's name and state of residence. Nakase-Richardson and colleagues (Nakase-Richardson, Yablon, Sherer, Nick, & Evans, 2009) demonstrated that these questions are of roughly equivalent difficulty and that these questions are most likely to be answered correctly by persons in early recovery from brain injury. So the patient is asked, "Is your name (correct name)?" and "Is your name (incorrect name)?" as well as "Do you live in (incorrect state)?" and "Do you live in (correct state)?" with multiple trials. The examiner should avoid having a predictable pattern of correct yes/no responses and should be alert to patient fatigue. Once reliable yes/no responses for these questions are achieved, it is reasonable to ask questions regarding whether or not the patient is in pain. It must be noted that reliability of yes/no responding can vary greatly across patients and within the same patient. Some patients may rarely give responses due to decreased level of arousal or poor initiation but be reliably accurate when they do give responses. Other patients may respond more often but achieve less than ideal consistency of response so that one cannot easily determine the accuracy of responses. For example, if a patient is correct 70% of the time on yes/no name questions, this is clearly above chance but perhaps not sufficiently accurate for one to trust responses to pain questions. Other patients may readily respond but show a marked bias to respond "yes" to almost all questions or, more rarely, "no" to almost all questions. Clearly, these responses cannot be relied upon.

The relative difficulty of yes/no questions about pain is not known, but given the strong salience of pain it is intuitive that such questions should be easy and that consistent yes/no responding should be achievable for these questions if it is achievable for any questions. The examiner should be aware that accuracy of yes/no responding may fluctuate due to fatigue, level of arousal, inattention, boredom, agitation, and other factors. It may be helpful to associate yes/no responses to pain questions with other possible behavioral indications of conscious awareness of pain such as facial expression, protection of a limb, shifting position, etc. However, these behaviors may have equivocal interpretation in confused and restless patients (see Chapter 3).

Persons who can give yes/no responses are at least in the MCS and those who can give consistently accurate yes/no responses have emerged from the MCS. It is possible that some patients in the MCS can respond with good, if not perfect, accuracy to highly salient questions such as name and pain questions even though they are not consistently accurate on the situational orientation questions used on the CRS-R. While persons who do not show functional object use or consistently respond accurately to situational orientation questions as specified in the case definition of emergence from the MCS (Giacino et al., 2002) are technically still minimally conscious, we believe that most clinicians concur that persons with consistent accuracy for name and state questions have emerged from the MCS.

Assessing persons in the post-traumatic confusional state

Persons who have emerged from unconsciousness lasting more than a few minutes enter a confusional state, or delirium. Others may also manifest a confusional state, but it is possible that some patients with brief disturbance of consciousness may not manifest a full confusional state though even these patients will likely have evidence of a period of amnesia with continued distractibility or other evidence of attentional disturbance. In persons with TBI, the confusional state is characterized by a global disturbance of attentional functions and is labeled the post-traumatic confusional state (PTCS; Stuss et al., 1999). In their pioneering work on this topic, Stuss and colleagues demonstrated the relative difficulty of simple attentional and memory tasks for persons in PTCS and demonstrated that recovery of the ability to perform such tasks follows a somewhat predictable pattern. PTCS can be considered to be a type of disordered consciousness in which the patient has partial awareness of the self and the environment but is often unable to successfully integrate this awareness due to marked impairment of attention and, perhaps, to level of arousal.

Sherer and colleagues (Sherer, Nakase-Thompson, Yablon, & Gontkovsky, 2005; Sherer, Yablon, & Nakase-Richardson, 2009; Sherer, Yablon, Nakase-Richardson, & Nick, 2008) extended Stuss and colleagues' work by identifying other key aspects of PTCS. Sherer and colleagues argue that key manifestations of PTCS are disorientation, cognitive impairment (actually impairment of simple attentional abilities, as demonstrated by Stuss and colleagues), fluctuation in clinical presentation, restlessness or agitation, nighttime sleep disturbance, decreased daytime arousal, and psychotic-type symptoms. Sherer and colleagues have provided diagnostic criteria and arbitrary cutoffs for mild, moderate, and severe confusion. Their work describes the typical course of recovery from confusion.

While the work of Stuss and Sherer's groups is specific to TBI, clinical experience suggests that similar findings are seen in persons emerging from MCS due to other causes (e.g., anoxia, stroke). While this literature has not investigated the relevance of PTCS to patient ability to provide accurate communication regarding perceived pain, it is reasonable to expect that persons in PTCS may not be able to accurately report pain. The most ubiquitous manifestation of PTCS is fluctuation in clinical presentation (Sherer et al., 2005). Persons in PTCS may be able to give accurate information regarding presence of pain at some exams but not others due to fluctuation in level of arousal, restlessness, and/or distractibility. Many persons in PTCS will be able to indicate the location and nature of their pain, but this ability may also fluctuate due to an excessive emotional response, agitation, or distractibility. Virtually all persons in PTCS will have substantial impairment of memory due to underlying memory disorder, inattention, or both. For this reason, it is unlikely that an accurate assessment of pain history can be obtained. Finally, persons in PTCS often show some evidence of aphasic-like speech, such as paraphasias, and may show possible signs of lack of initiation at times. These problems can also limit pain assessment.

When attempting to assess pain in the confused patient, it is important to structure the setting and interaction to maximize the likelihood of accurate responding. Given the distractibility of confused patients, it is desirable to have a quiet environment with limited visual stimulation. Persons other than the interviewer should be behind the patient or, at least, to his or her side. Only one person should address the patient, and this person should be directly in front of the patient or to the more intact side if the patient has findings indicating a possible visual field defect or neglect. Questions should be asked in a calm conversational tone that indicates genuine concern for the patient. This approach may engage the patient in a social interaction mode of communication, given the powerful pull for this type of interaction for most persons. A more clinical, matter-of-fact tone may be less likely to engage this social response. The calm tone of voice may help to minimize the restlessness or excessive emotional responding (i.e., lability) that can occur in these patients. Agitated or labile patients may respond to repeated encouragement to calm down if this encouragement is spoken in a soft, calm tone, but on other occasions it will be necessary to discontinue the interview and return later. Given the degree of memory impairment and attentional disturbance seen in some patients, it may be possible to reapproach the patient only a few minutes later and obtain a more productive response.

Some patients who are hypoaroused will benefit from some stimulation to enhance their level of arousal and responsiveness. We generally use shoulder massage with increasing firmness as needed to enhance arousal level. For some patients, it may be necessary to continue firm massage throughout the interview to maintain responsiveness. This massage is a less intense form of the Arousal Facilitation Protocol described by Giacino and Kalmar for the CRS-R (Giacino & Kalmar, 2004).

As noted above, some confused patients will be able to identify the location and nature of pain in addition to indicating whether or not they are experiencing pain. In general, we recommend that the patient be asked to state the body part that is in pain and also point to the body part that is in pain. These requests should be made more than once, a few minutes apart, during the interview. Consistency, between naming and pointing to painful locations and between responses at different points in the interview, provides some reassurance that responses can be trusted. Body schematics can be used to help patients with localizing pain, but until repeatable accuracy is demonstrated one should not trust left/right discrimination or even front/back discrimination. Similarly, when assessing the nature of pain, it is helpful to pair a verbal label with having the patient point to a schematic representing the type of pain (e.g., throbbing, burning, aching). Consistency between the verbal label and the schematic identified enhances confidence. Again, there should be multiple trials to demonstrate that responses are consistent.

To assess pain severity, it is reasonable to use visual analog scales as used with nonconfused patients. As with localization of pain, one should use multiple trials to ensure consistent responding. A complementary strategy is to have the patient relate the current pain intensity to painful experiences in the remote past. Even confused patients may recall emotionally salient experiences from the remote past so that one may be able to obtain a menu of painful experiences from the past. So then a patient reporting arm pain could be asked to compare the intensity of the pain to the pain felt when he or she broke his or her arm in the third grade. This is an unvalidated procedure that should be used only with caution to augment more standard approaches, such as when the patient is inconsistent in pointing to responses on a visual analog pain scale. As noted above, given impaired attention and memory, it is unlikely to be useful to ask the patient to compare pain from one day to the next or to report on the beneficial effect of pain therapies such as medications. A more fruitful approach to judging response to therapies will be to observe the frequency and intensity of pain behaviors as well as the patient's degree of participation in therapy activities.

Memory impairment and pain assessment

Once the confusional state resolves, and assuming the absence of aphasia or a marked disorder of initiation, the patient will generally be able to report at most examinations whether or not he or she is in pain as well as the location and nature of pain. Still, persons in early recovery from severe brain injury or illness may show substantial fluctuation in cognitive and behavioral functioning even after confusion resolves. Consequently, accuracy of reporting may vary, though this variation will be much less than for patients in a confusional state. Even when reporting in the moment is accurate, persistent memory impairment may complicate pain assessment (Sherer & Madison, 2005). Ability to accurately report on the evolution of pain and response to pain therapies depends on recall of earlier status or recall of self-reports of this earlier status. Memory impairment due to a traumatic injury or stroke is likely to have a recovering course, though the course after anoxia may be less favorable. Introspection of a subjective experience such as the severity of pain in the moment and comparing this severity to a previous experience poses substantial cognitive demand, particularly given the strong affective component of pain response in some persons. One could question whether even persons with no cognitive impairment can perform this task with great accuracy.

Interviewers should seek to minimize the impact of memory impairment on pain evaluations in persons recovering from brain injury. Pain severity is commonly rated on a 10-point scale. Ratings can be plotted on a graph so that the patient can see the pattern of ratings from previous days and compare the degree of pain experienced on the current day to earlier days. As the patient's memory improves, the patient can be asked to recall the previous rating before being shown the chart. As suggested above for confused patients, the patient can be asked to compare the current level of pain to a reference level of pain that the patient experienced in the remote past. As remote memory is generally relatively spared, there is a reasonable chance that this approach will work in the patient with fairly isolated recent memory impairment and nonconfused patients will be more accurate, in general, than confused patients.

Assessing persons with aphasia

Aphasia is an acquired impairment of language processing (Albert & Helm-Estabrooks, 1998). It affects expressive language as well as language comprehension in virtually all affected persons, though some may be thought to have relatively preserved comprehension in the face of more severe expressive deficits. In our experience, assessment with standardized tests usually reveals greater than expected impairment of comprehension in those thought to have preservation of comprehension based on clinical observation. Aphasia usually affects spoken and written language, though in some cases one modality may be affected more than another. Key issues in assessment of aphasia include whether speech is fluent or dysfluent, presence of paraphasias (word substitutions) and/ or jargon (neologisms), degree of impairment of naming (anomia), and degree of impairment of repetition. There are a number of classification schemas for aphasia, though many patients have mixed syndromes. Some degree of aphasia may be seen in virtually any patient with a DOC who recovers to a responsive state. However severe, persistent aphasia is much more common after major left hemisphere stroke than after right hemisphere stroke, TBI, or anoxia. Aphasia complicates assessment of consciousness and degree of confusion due to its general effect on patient response to many behavioral assessment techniques (Majerus, Bruno, Schnackers, Giacino, & Laureys, 2009).

Many patients show some evidence of aphasia, such as paraphasic substitutions during the confusional state, that may resolve once the patient is no longer confused. Patients thought to have poor initiation during the confusional state may be found to have aphasia as they improve in other areas of neurologic function. Neuroimaging can be useful in assessing the likelihood of a persistent aphasia in patients in early recovery. Possible indications of underlying aphasia in persons in early recovery include: (1) halting speech, (2) word substitutions,

(3) use of non-words, (4) occasional empty speech in a social context (e.g., responding "Fine, how are you?" to a question about how the patient is doing) with little or no initiation of speech in other contexts, (5) inability to repeat words, (6) inability or severe difficulty in naming common objects, (7) marked dissociation between ability to perform a simple command when given a demonstration along with the command as compared to when no demonstration is provided, (8) answering yes to virtually all questions when cued by a head nod from the interviewer and answering no to virtually all questions when cued by a headshake, and others.

Marked aphasia is likely to be associated with impairment of other cognitive abilities, though this can be difficult to demonstrate as most cognitive tests rely on verbal responses or, at least, on the ability to comprehend and respond to verbal instructions. Some persons with aphasia will not attempt to initiate any communication, perhaps due to frustration or learned disuse. All of these factors can make assessment of pain in the aphasic patient most challenging. If the patient does not give reliable, comprehensible responses to verbally presented questions, written presentation can be attempted – though this is likely to fail as well. One can try symbols representing burning, stabbing, aching, etc. to see if the patient can associate these with bodily sensations. Even here it is difficult to imagine a procedure for introducing these stimuli that would not require at least some minimal language comprehension. Fortunately, aphasia severity is variable so a degree of communication will be possible with some patients. If aphasia is so severe as to limit any response to examination, one must rely on observation of pain behaviors such as shifting positions, limb protection, facial expression, avoidance of activities, etc.

Patients with marked disturbance of motivation

Some degree of decreased motivation is common in patients with bilateral medial brain lesions or in those with large lesions. Generally this is manifested as decreased initiation so that, with cuing, the patient may be able to complete complex behavioral acts. In some cases, verbal cuing is not sufficient and the patient may require a physical cue, such as a gentle lift under the arm to come to standing. When the patient is vegetative or even minimally conscious, it may be very difficult to dissociate a motivational disorder from the DOC. As patients progress, motivational disorders may masquerade as decreased level of arousal or may be interpreted by others as a sign of depression. While motivational disorders may not be common, as they generally require bilateral lesions (Giacino, Fins, Laureys, & Schiff, 2014), they should be considered as a possible explanation for poor communication and/or low levels of activity in a patient who seems to have capacity for a higher level of functioning or who occasionally performs fairly complex behaviors before returning to a largely inactive state. If possible, one should consider obtaining MRI imaging to assist with this diagnosis. Persons with dense disorders of motivation may show almost no spontaneous movement or communication and are diagnosed with akinetic mutism (Giacino et al., 2014). Fortunately, motivational disorders occur on a continuum and profoundly severe disorders are rare. More commonly, the patient shows occasional or limited behavior. An underlying motivational disorder is a possible cause of persistent MCS.

Since motivational disorders are often associated with damage to dopaminergic pathways and targets, treatment with dopaminergic agents may be helpful for some patients. Behavioral approaches to treatment involve prompting. For verbal behavior, one may begin a common saying or sequence to see if the patient will finish it. So the interviewer might say, "Three strikes and you are ___" in hope that the patient will provide the word "out." Alternatively, the interviewer might say, "The colors in the United States flag are red, white, and ___." For physical acts such as feeding or grooming, the clinician can use a hand-over-hand prompt to start the act. It is challenging to translate these prompts to some type of assessment of pain. One might try, "My arm hurts right here (pointing to a place on the arm in an exaggerated gesture). Where do you hurt?" Similarly, one might try, "I hurt this much (holding hands wide apart), but yesterday I only hurt this much (holding hands close together). Show me how much you hurt." One would hope to have multiple similar responses to increase confidence in the meaning of a response, but obtaining even one response may be a challenge with some patients. In such cases, accurate assessment of level, location, and type of subjective pain may be impossible. Failure to respond would not necessarily indicate that the patient is not experiencing pain. As with other patients with low levels of responsiveness, one can observe for pain behavior. Unfortunately, an amotivational patient may be less likely to show these behaviors as well.

Summary

Patients with severe DOC cannot participate in routine clinical assessment of pain. However, as patients with DOC improve it is important to consider additional factors that may limit accurate assessment of pain despite emerging consciousness. That is, consciousness is necessary for accurate reporting of pain but it is far from sufficient. Patients who cannot provide any useful information about painful conditions via interview must be evaluated through physical examination and behavioral observation. Physical examination may provide hypotheses as to the source of pain, and observation of behaviors indicative of nociception or pain (e.g., grimaces, guarding) may help confirm these hypotheses. Standardized observational measures of pain behaviors exist for some patient populations and those specifically for patients with DOC are in various stages of development (see Chapter 3). For patients who can provide some information about pain but are behaviorally variable and unreliable, it may be possible to increase the confidence in their reporting by asking related questions on multiple occasions and basing the conclusion on the pattern of responding rather than on the reply to a single question. In the early post-injury period, however, consciousness, the impairments that complicate assessment of consciousness, and conditions producing pain may all be undergoing rapid evolution. Thus, the clinician must view each assessment conclusion as tentative and must be vigilant for clinical changes that demand reassessment.

Acknowledgment

The authors would like to thank Dr. Miriam Segal for consultation on the clinical cases presented.

Notes

1 **John Whyte**, MD, PhD, FACRM, is Director at Moss Rehabilitation Research Institute in Philadelphia. He is a staff physiatrist for Einstein Practice Plan and has teaching appointments at Jefferson Medical College and Temple University School of Medicine.
2 **Mark Sherer**, PhD, ABPP, FACRM, is Senior Scientist and Director of Research at TIRR Memorial Hermann, Houston, TX. He is a clinical professor of Physical Medicine and Rehabilitation at Baylor College of Medicine and the University of Texas Medical School at Houston.

References

Albert, M.L., & Helm-Estabrooks, N. (1998). Diagnosis and treatment of aphasia: part 1. *Journal of the American Medical Association*, 259(Feb 19), 1043–1047.

Barrett, A.M., & Foundas, A.L. (2004). Apraxia. In M. Rizzo & P.J. Eslinger (Eds.), *Principles and Practice of Behavioral Neurology and Neuropsychology* (pp. 409–422). Philadelphia: Saunders/Churchill/Livingstone/Mosby.

Buxbaum, L.J., Ferraro, M.K., Veramonti, T., Farne, A., Whyte, J., Ladavas, E., . . . Coslet, H.B. (2004). Hemispatial neglect: subtypes, neuroanatomy, and disability. *Neurology*, 62, 749–765.

Celesia, G., & Brigell, M. (2005). Cortical blindness and visual agnosia. In Celesia, G., & Brigell, M. (Eds.), *Disorders of Visual Processing: Handbook of Clinical Neurophysiology* (Vol. 5, pp. 429–440). Philadelphia: Elsevier.

Giacino, J., Ashwal, S., Childs, N., Cranford, R., Jennett, B., Katz, D., . . . Zasler, N. (2002). The minimally conscious state: definition and diagnostic criteria. *Neurology*, 58, 349–353.

Giacino, J.T., Fins, J.J., Laureys, S., & Schiff, N.D. (2014). Disorders of consciousness after acquired brain injury: the state of the science. *Nature Reviews: Neurology*, 10, 99–114.

Giacino, J.T., & Kalmar, K. (2004). *CRS-R Coma Recovery Scale-Revised: Administration and Scoring Guidelines*. Edison, NJ: Center for Head Injuries.

Giacino, J.T., Kalmar, K., & Whyte, J. (2004). The JFK Coma Recovery Scale-Revised: measurement characteristics and diagnostic utility. *Archives of Physical Medicine and Rehabilitation*, 85(12), 2020–2029.

Giacino, J., & Whyte, J. (2005). The vegetative and minimally conscious states: current knowledge and remaining questions. *Journal of Head Trauma Rehabilitation*, 20(1), 30–50.

Latronico, N., & Bolton, C.F. (2011). Critical illness polyneuropathy and myopathy: a major cause of muscle weakness and paralysis. *[Review] Lancet Neurology*, 10(10), 931–941.

Majerus, S., Bruno, M.A., Schnackers, C., Giacino, J.T., & Laureys, S. (2009). The problem of aphasia in the assessment of consciousness in brain-damaged patients. *Progress in Brain Reseach*, 177, 49–61.

Nagaratnam, N., Nagaratnam, K., Ng, K., & Diu, P. (2004). Akinetic mutism following stroke. *Journal of Clinical Neuroscience*, 11(1), 25–30.

Nakase-Richardson, R., Yablon, S. A., Sherer, M., Nick, T. G., & Evans, C. C. (2009). Emergence from the minimally conscious state: insights from evaluation of posttraumatic confusion. *Neurology*, 73, 1120–1126.

National Institutes of Health. (2008). What causes aphasia? In Voice, Speech and Language: Aphasia. Retrieved from http://www.nidcd.nih.gov/health/voice/pages/aphasia.aspx#causes

Rappaport, M., Hall, K. M., Hopkins, K., Belleza, T., & Cope, D. N. (1982). Disability Rating Scale for severe head trauma: coma to community. *Archives of Physical Medicine and Rehabilitation*, 63, 118–123.

Seel, R. T., Sherer, M., Whyte, J., Katz, D. I., Giacino, J. T., Shapiro, A., . . . Zasler, N. (2010). Assessment scales for disorders of consciousness: evidence-based recommendations for clinical practice and research. *Archives of Physical Medicine and Rehabilitation*, 91(12), 1795–1813.

Sherer, M., & Madison, C. F. (2005). Moderate and severe traumatic brain injury. In G. L. Larrabee (Ed.), *Forensic Neuropsychology: A Scientific Approach* (pp. 237–270). New York: Oxford University Press.

Sherer, M., Nakase-Thompson, R., Yablon, S. A., & Gontkovsky, S. T. (2005). Multidimensional assessment of acute confusion after traumatic brain injury. *Archives of Physical Medicine and Rehabilitation*, 86(5), 896–904.

Sherer, M., Yablon, S. A., & Nakase-Richardson, R. (2009). Patterns of recovery of posttraumatic confusional state in neurorehabilitation admissions after traumatic brain injury. *Archives of Physical Medicine and Rehabilitation*, 90(10), 1749–1754.

Sherer, M., Yablon, S. A., Nakase-Richardson, R., & Nick, T. G. (2008). Effect of severity of post-traumatic confusion and its constituent symptoms on outcome after traumatic brain injury. *Archives of Physical Medicine and Rehabilitation*, 89(1), 42–47.

Smith, S. M., Hunsinger, M., McKeown, A., Parkhurst, M., Allen, R., Kopko, S., & Dworkin, R. H. (2015). Quality of pain intensity assessment reporting: ACTTION systematic review and recommendations. *Journal of Pain*, Advance online publication.

Stuss, D. T., Binns, M. A., Carruth, F. G., Levine, B., Brandys, C. E., Moulton, R. J., . . . Schwartz, M. F. (1999). The acute period of recovery from traumatic brain injury: posttraumatic amnesia or posttraumatic confusional state? *Neurosurgery*, 90(4), 635–643.

Van Erp, W. S., Lavrijsen, J. C., Vos, P. E., Bor, H., Laureys, S., & Koopman, R. T. (2015). The vegetative state: prevalence, misdiagnosis, and treatment limitation. *Journal of the American Medical Directors Association*, 85(1), e9–e85.

Whyte, J., & DiPasquale, M. (1995). Assessment of vision and visual attention in minimally responsive brain injured patients. *Archives of Physical Medicine and Rehabilitation*, 76(9), 804–810.

Whyte, J., DiPasquale, M., & Vaccaro, M. (1999). Assessment of command-following in minimally conscious brain injured patients. *Archives of Physical Medicine and Rehabilitation*, 80, 1–8.

Whyte, J., Laborde, A., & DiPasquale, M. C. (1999). Assessment and treatment of the vegetative and minimally conscious patient. In M. Rosenthal, E. R. Griffith, J. S. Kreutzer & B. Pentland (Eds.), *Rehabilitation of the Adult and Child with Traumatic Brain Injury* (3rd ed., Vol. 25, pp. 435–452). Philadelphia: F. A. Davis.

Whyte, J., Ponsford, J., Watanabe, T., & Hart, T. (2010). Traumatic brain injury. In J. A. DeLisa (Ed.), *Physical Medicine and Rehabilitation: Principles and Practice* (Vol. 1, pp. 575–624). Philadelphia: Lippincott, Williams & Wilkins.

Yeomans, J. S., & Frankland, P. W. (1996). The acoustic startle reflex: neurons and connections. *Brain Research Reviews*, 21, 301–314.

5 Using paraclinical assessments to detect consciousness and communicate with severely brain-injured patients

Camille Chatelle[1] and Damien Lesenfants[2]

Abbreviations

BCI	brain-computer interface
DOC	disorders of consciousness
ECoG	electrocorticography
EEG	electroencephalography
EMG	electromyography
fMRI	functional magnetic resonance imaging
fNIRS	functional near-infrared spectroscopy
LIS	locked-in syndrome
MCS	minimally conscious state
VS/UWS	vegetative state/unresponsive wakefulness syndrome

Introduction

Motor disability is a prevalent challenge for clinicians working with severely brain-injured patients in terms of diagnosis, care, and rehabilitation (Cruse et al., 2011; Monti et al., 2010; Owen et al., 2006; Schnakers et al., 2009). As discussed in Chapters 1 and 4, behavioral assessment, which is highly dependent on motor abilities, remains the traditional way to evaluate consciousness (i.e., command-following and/or communication) in these patients. However, recent studies reported command-specific changes in signals recorded with electroencephalography (EEG) or functional magnetic resonance imaging (fMRI) in about 18% of severely brain-injured patients who were diagnosed as unconscious at the bedside (Chatelle et al., 2012; Cruse et al., 2011; Goldfine, Victor, Conte, Bardin, & Schiff, 2011a; Lulé et al., 2013; Monti et al., 2010; Schnakers et al., 2009; Schnakers et al., 2008b). These findings had a major impact on the way we think about noncommunicative patients, in particular in the context of treatment and pain assessment. Indeed, the idea that such patients may be able to communicate about their feelings and provide information about their level of pain using their brain activity is at the same time upsetting and exciting. However, current methods are often dependent on residual motor preservation (Combaz et al., 2013; Kubler & Birbaumer, 2008;

Piccione et al., 2006) and/or require time-consuming user training (Birbaumer, 2006; Kubler & Birbaumer, 2008; Neuper, Müller-Putz, Kubler, Birbaumer, & Pfurtscheller, 2003), all of which prevent them from being used for detecting command-following and communication in this population. Furthermore, the high rate (22–94%) of false negatives (patients who show command-following at the bedside but who are not detected with the system; see also Chatelle, Lesenfants, Guller, Laureys, & Noirhomme, 2015; Monti et al., 2010; Schnakers et al., 2008b) and the issue of false positives (patients detected by the system as showing command-following who are actually unconscious; Cruse et al., 2013; Goldfine et al., 2013) highlight the current need to develop more reliable tools for this population. The availability of reliable systems would have a significant impact on providing care such as treatment (in particular, for pain and anxiety) and rehabilitation, as well as on quality of life (Kubler, Mushahwar, Hochberg, & Donoghue, 2006).

In this chapter, we will review the studies on paraclinical assessments for detecting response to command and communication in patients with disorders of consciousness (DOC), taking into account the number of patients showing command-following with the system and how many of them were able to follow a command at the bedside that could not be detected by the system (i.e., false negatives). The false positive rate should also be considered but will not be discussed here as it is difficult to determine the level of consciousness of patients diagnosed as being unconscious but who show response to command with a paraclinical assessment. We will also highlight the main challenges that will need to be overcome in future research.

Paraclinical assessment for detecting command-following and establishing communication in DOC

Cortically-based techniques

The first study showing the possibility of detecting response to command using an active task was conducted by Owen et al. in 2006, when a patient diagnosed as being in a vegetative state/unresponsive wakefulness syndrome (VS/UWS) was able to follow the instruction to "imagine playing tennis" and "imagine walking through her house" during an fMRI session (Owen et al., 2006). The paradigm consisted of several sessions of mental imagery followed by a resting period, both lasting 30 seconds. Similar brain activation as compared to that in healthy volunteers was observed for both tasks. In addition, the patient behaviorally evolved into minimally conscious state (MCS) a few months after the study. In a follow-up study (Monti et al., 2010) including 54 patients (see Table 5.1), five patients (four VS/UWS) showed the ability to willfully modulate their brain activity according to the task. One of them was also able to answer simple questions (e.g., "Is your father's name Alexander?") using one task for "yes" and the other for "no." However, out of 18 patients who showed command-following at the bedside, only one could be identified with the system (false negative rate: 94%).

This study was the first to bring hope for improving diagnosis and communication in this population. The paradigm was also used more recently to try to establish binary communication with a patient who had been in a VS/UWS for more than 12 years (Fernández-Espejo & Owen, 2013). In this study, the patient was asked basic autobiographical questions as well as semantic, orientation, new knowledge, and personal preference questions. Interestingly, the researchers also asked him questions relative to his quality of life (e.g., "Are you in pain?"). It has to be noted that the patient did not respond on every occasion; sometimes no significant activity could be observed, which suggested a lack of attention, motivation, or will on that particular day. This highlights the current main limitation to applying these methods in clinical settings and to interpreting the findings to drive decisions in care and treatments.

Further studies were conducted to improve the sensitivity of paraclinical assessments and our understanding of the observed phenomena Bardin et al. (2011) investigated the use of a different imagery task instructing patients to imagine themselves swimming or playing tennis, using a similar protocol to the one used by Owen et al. (2006) and Monti et al. (2010). They reported three out of six patients who were able to follow commands with the system. However, two out of the five patients able to follow commands at the bedside could not be identified with the system (false negative rate: 40%). Similarly, using an active task in fMRI (counting a target word in an auditory sequence of non-targets words), Monti et al. (2009) reported preserved working memory abilities in a MCS patient exceeding that which could be observed with standard behavioral assessment. This patient was able to follow a command and communicate non-functionally at the bedside. In yet another study, three patients were instructed to either count the occurrences of a target word ("yes" or "no") or simply relax and passively listen to a sequence of "yes" and "no" presented within a sequence of numbers (Naci & Owen, 2013). Command-following could be detected in all of the patients, and two patients were able to focus their attention to communicate correct answers to two binary ("yes" or "no") questions (e.g., "Are you in a supermarket?" or "Is your name Steven?").

These first studies showing response to command in patients with DOC were conducted using fMRI, a technique that has many limitations that prevent it from being applied in a clinical setting. First, ferrous metallic implants are a contraindication to MRI, preventing many patients from undergoing this procedure. Even if implants are nonferrous, metal in the head can cause significant image artifact, making analysis of the results difficult or impossible. Second, fMRI is sensitive to motion, which can result from reflexive movement in the scanner, general restlessness, or decreased patient cooperation. Images that are affected by significant motion artifact cannot be interpreted. Finally, many clinical settings do not have access to MRI because it is an expensive technique to implement and it requires personnel with expertise to process the data. These exclusion criteria have been observed during the European FP7 DECODER project (Deployment of Brain-Computer Interfaces for the Detection of Consciousness in Non-Responsive Patients). Out of the 169 patients with DOC elected for a fMRI active sport/navigation paradigm at the Centre Hospitalier Universitaire de Liège (Belgium) during the three years of the DECODER project, only 60 yielded active paradigm data that were interpretable, mainly because of reflexive head motion in the scanner.

Given these limitations, EEG may be better suited for assessing patients with DOC as it is not contraindicated by metallic implants and is less sensitive to motion. EEG is also relatively inexpensive, compact, and accessible in most clinical settings, so it can be readily deployed at the bedside and used for repetitive assessments. In recent years, researchers have been developing EEG-based tasks to assess response to command in DOC.

As suggested by fMRI studies, imagination of movement may be a reasonable method to supplement observation of actual movement during standard behavioral assessment. EEG studies have shown that motor imagery is associated with a power decrease (event-related desynchronization) in the sensorimotor or mu-rhythm (8–15 Hz; Neuper, Scherer, Reiner, & Pfurtscheller, 2005; Pfurtscheller, Neuper, Flotzinger, & Pregenzer, 1997), focused in the motor region that is implicated in the movement being imagined (Pfurtscheller & Lopes da Silva, 1999). Goldfine and colleagues (Goldfine, Victor, Conte, Bardin, & Schiff, 2011b) recorded EEG from three patients showing command-following at the bedside while they were involved in motor imagery and spatial navigation tasks. All of the patients demonstrated the capacity to generate mental imagery on the same tasks on independent fMRI studies. Goldfine and colleagues showed evidence of significant differences in EEG activity between the two imagery tasks in two patients (however, results were not stable between the two runs; false negative rate: 33%).

In another study from Cruse et al., motor imagery tasks were investigated in 16 VS/UWS patients (Cruse et al., 2011) and in 23 MCS patients (Cruse et al., 2012a). Eight patients (three VS/UWS, five MCS) were able to voluntary control their brain activity in response to a command ("imagine squeezing your right hand" or "imagine moving all your toes"). Out of 15 patients showing command-following at the bedside, 13 could not be identified by the system (false negative rate: 87%).

However, other studies have suggested that motor imagery cannot be reliably used and interpreted in severely motor-disabled patients (Bai et al., 2008; Kubler et al., 2005). Instead of motor imagery, Nijboer et al. recommended the use of the P3 response in patients with severe motor impairment (Nijboer, Birbaumer, & Kubler, 2010). The P3 response is a positive deflection in the EEG appearing around 200–500 milliseconds following a target stimulus. Its advantage is that it can be elicited by meaningful stimuli and requires a limited working memory load from the patient. Schnakers et al. proposed using an auditory P3 for detecting command-following using EEG (Schnakers et al., 2008b). They asked 22 patients to count the number of times a name (the subject's own name or an unfamiliar name) was presented within an auditory sequence of random names (Schnakers et al., 2008b). Results showed that five out of 14 MCS patients showed significantly greater P3 responses when actively counting the occurrence of their own name as compared to when they were only passively listening to it. Four additional MCS patients showed a response only when they were asked to count an unfamiliar name as compared to passive listening. These results suggest that fluctuation of vigilance may play a role in task performance in this population. The eight VS/UWS patients did not show any response to the active counting task. The same paradigm has been used in a patient behaviorally diagnosed as being comatose, who showed a significant difference between the passive and the active task (Schnakers et al., 2009). Following this finding, this patient was reassessed and diagnosed with complete locked-in syndrome (LIS; see Chapter 6 for more details on research in LIS). This extreme case illustrates the clinical utility of paraclinical tools as a supplement to behavioral assessment. Using this paradigm, two out of eight patients showing command-following at bedside could not be detected with the system (false negative rate: 25%). Similar results have been replicated in a recent study including 11 patients with DOC, eight VS/UWS, and three MCS (Risetti et al., 2013).

Finally, extensive research on attention involving healthy subjects has suggested that the P3 response should be deconstructed into separable subcomponents represented by the P3a and P3b. The early frontally centered novelty P3a would be associated with exogenous attention, triggered by stimulus novelty ("bottom-up") that may be task-irrelevant, whereas the later parietally focused P3b, on the other hand, is seen as a marker of volitional endogenous attention to task-relevant targets necessary for consolidation into working memory and for conscious access ("top down") (Polich, 2007). Chennu et al. (2013) developed a paradigm aiming to engender exogenous or endogenous attention (i.e., P3a and P3b EEG response), respectively, in response to a pair of word stimuli presented auditorily among distracters. Among the 21 patients included in the study, none of the seven patients showing command-following at the bedside generated a P3b (false negative rate: 100%), three patients generated only early nondiscriminative responses to targets (including two patients showing command-following at the bedside – false negative rate: 71%), and one patient in VS/UWS generated both a P3a and a P3b response. Interestingly, 20 of these patients were also administered the fMRI paradigm developed by Owen et al. (Monti et al., 2010; Owen et al., 2006). In six patients in whom no discernible P3a/P3b response could be elicited, a response to command using fMRI tennis imagery task could be detected. This discrepancy may be explained by fluctuation of arousal or heterogeneity in terms of the preservation of specific neural structures and the cognitive resources available (Gibson et al., 2014). It also suggests that the level of difficulty required by this attention task is too high to enable a good rate of detection of conscious patients. However, the VS/UWS patient who showed P3a/P3b responses did also show a response to command with the fMRI, supporting the idea that the presence of a P3a and P3b may highlight a well-preserved volitional attention process.

All the methods presented above used active tasks that are usually used for controlling brain-computer interfaces (BCI). However, the difference between a standard active paradigm and a BCI is the interaction between the system (computer, machine, etc.) and the user that allows a communication between the brain and the external environment (Wolpaw, Birbaumer, McFarland, Pfurtscheller, & Vaughan, 2002). A BCI offers a person the possibility to control a system with his own brain activity (Sellers & Donchin, 2006; Sellers, Kubler, & Donchin, 2006). A specific algorithm translates the task-related brain features into commands that represent the user's intent and provides feedback. As illustrated in Figure 5.1, modifications of brain activity due to a task/stimulus can be recorded using fMRI, fNIRS, EEG, or ECoG. These neural data are preprocessed before discriminative features are extracted. Machine learning techniques are then used to train classifiers to detect statistical patterns in the features that are reliably associated with prespecified (supervised) volitional states of the user. The trained classifier is then used to classify new features corresponding to states now selected by the user to communicate choices. Finally, the result of the classification is fed back to the user to help her train herself in the use of the BCI and to help clinicians detect a response to command or communicate with the patient.

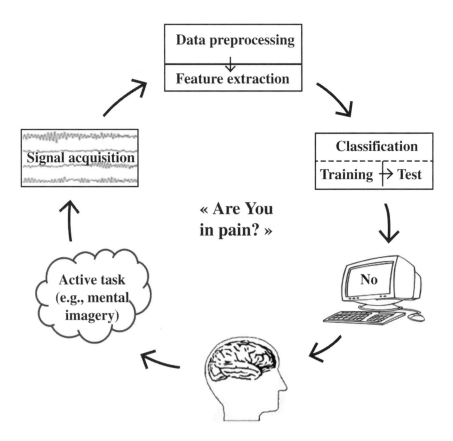

Figure 5.1 A typical brain-computer interface.

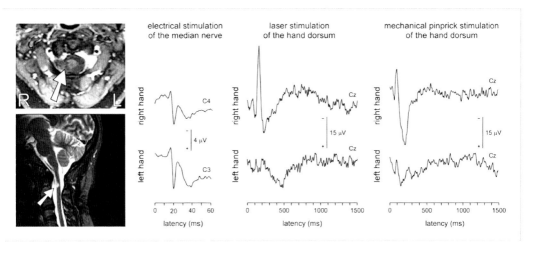

Figure 2.1 Nociceptive and non-nociceptive somatosensory-evoked potentials recorded in a patient presenting with thermal and pinprick hypoesthesia of the left hemibody following the surgical removal of a spinal neurinoma at level C1-C2 (adapted from Iannetti et al. 2013).

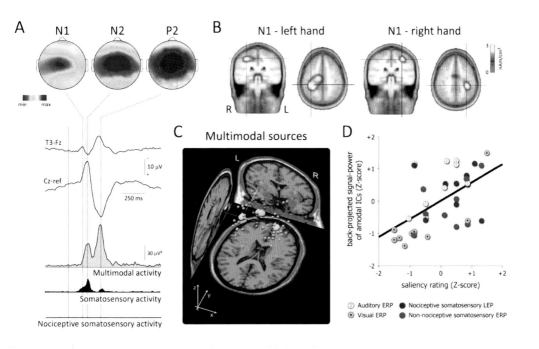

Figure 2.2 **A**. Blind-source separation of nociceptive ERPs elicited by short pulses of radiant heat delivered to the hand dorsum using an infrared laser. **B**. Source analyses of the N1 wave of nociceptive ERPs elicited by stimulation of the left- and right-hand dorsum. **C**. Source analysis of the multimodal activity constituting the N2 and P2 waves. **D**. Correlation between the magnitude of this multimodal activity (Y-axis) and perceived stimulus salience (X-axis) (adapted from Mouraux et al., 2010, and Valentini et al., 2012).

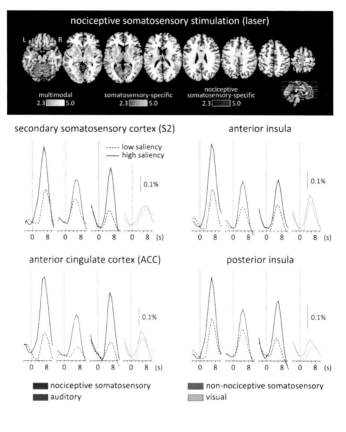

Figure 2.3 Overlap between the fMRI BOLD responses elicited by transient nociceptive stimuli and transient non-nociceptive somatosensory, auditory, and visual stimuli applied to or around the right foot (adapted from Mouraux, Diukova, Lee, Wise, & Iannetti, 2011a).

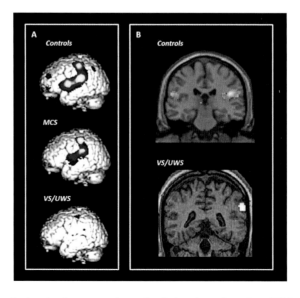

Figure 3.1 Cerebral activation to noxious stimulation in patients in a VS/UWS and in a MCS as compared to healthy controls (adapted from Chatelle et al., 2014).

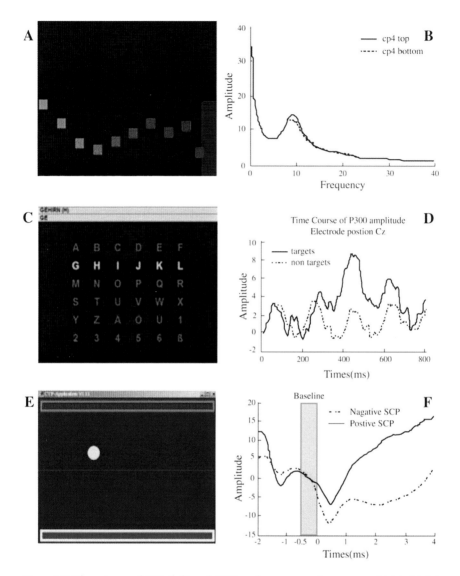

Figure 6.2 Three types of BCI (left) and EEG analyses averaged over several trials (right). **A**: Depicts the SMR-BCI as the patient moves the cursor (square) into the target (red block at the right bottom corner). **B**: Amplitude of the EEG as a function of frequency during cursor movement. **C**: Depicts P300-BCI 6×6 letter matrix. **D**: Course of EEG during letter selection. **E**: Depicts SCP-BCI as the patient moves the cursor (yellow dot) toward the target with the highlighted frame. **F**: Time course of the SCP amplitude separated by task requirement. (Figure from Kübler et al., 2008.)

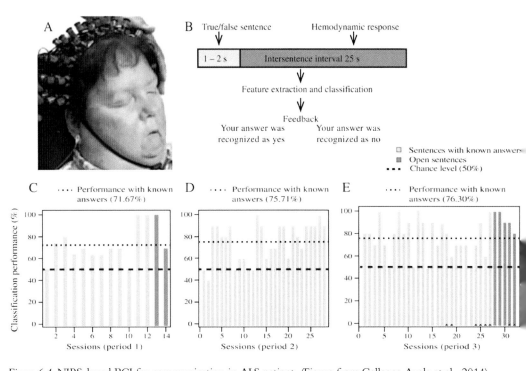

Figure 6.4 NIRS-based BCI for communication in ALS patient. (Figure from Gallegos-Ayala et al., 2014).

Note: **(A)** Brain oxygenation and deoxygenation changes in hemoglobin were recorded with an ETG-4000 Optical Topograph System (HitachiMedical Co., Tokyo, Japan) covering the sensorimotor cortex and temporal areas. The figure shows the patie with the NIRS sensors and receivers attached to her head. **(B)** The structure of sentences, as presented by the NIRS-based BC **(C)** Classification performance based on the questions with known answers in period 1, which consisted of 12 sessions spre over 14 days with 105 true and 95 false sentences. Sessions with questions requiring a known answer are blue. Sessions 13 and contained 20 open questions that are orange. **(D)** Classification performance of each session with known answers in period (28 sessions distributed across eight days with 140 true and 140 false sentences). **(E)** Classification performance of each session wi known answers in period 3 (27 sessions spread over two weeks with 135 true and 135 false sentences). Sessions 28 to 32 contained open questions. Sessions marked with a small black triangle consisted of sentences recorded with an unfamiliar voice; all oth sessions were recorded with the voice of the patient's husband. The classification results of the open sentences in periods 1 and were derived from the assumed correct answers the husband had noted before the sessions. The session sequence for sessions wi known answers follows the numbers below the respective bars. The sessions with open answers were interspersed in time betwe the sessions with known answers in period 3 but were moved to the end of the figure to underscore their importance. The char level is marked by a black horizontal line; the average performance level is marked in blue.

These commands can control effectors to select items such as words, images, or devices. Recent development has shown the usefulness of BCIs for controlling motor prosthesis and cursors, for providing a means of communication, and for accessing the Internet (Citi, Poli, Cinel, & Sepulveda, 2008; Hochberg et al., 2012; Hochberg et al., 2006; Lee, Ryu, Jolesz, Cho, & Yoo, 2009; Mugler, Ruf, Halder, Bensch, & Kler, 2010; Sellers, Vaughan, & Wolpaw, 2010; Yoo et al., 2004).

In the context of DOC, a BCI would allow clinicians to detect command-specific changes in brain signals as evidence of conscious thoughts. Then, if the patient is able to reproducibly follow a command using the system, the software and hardware can be extended to test communication. It is important to remember that the detection of response to command is the cornerstone in the determination of the correct state of consciousness, indicating a transition from the VS/UWS to the MCS. A functional communication illustrates an emergence from the MCS. A BCI may also help clinicians to detect patients with LIS in the acute stage, when the difficulty of recognizing unambiguous signs of consciousness often results in the diagnosis being delayed or even missed (Laureys et al., 2005).

A few studies have been conducted using BCI in patients with DOC. A study by Lulé et al. used a four-choice auditory-based paradigm for communication with three VS/UWS, 13 MCS, and two LIS patients (Lulé et al., 2013). After a training phase, each patient was asked to answer 10 questions by concentrating on repetitions of "yes" or "no" presented in a stream of different words (yes, no, stop, go). One LIS patient reached 79% offline accuracy, while the second patient showed accuracy at chance level. When using the system online, no patient could achieve performances allowing communication (i.e., >70% accuracy, Kubler & Birbaumer, 2008). As a result, neither of the two patients showing functional communication at the bedside could use the system to communicate with online feedback (false negative: 100%). However, the task assessed communication (the patient had to answer a series of questions), necessitating a higher level of cognitive functioning than basic one-step commands. This could explain the very low performances observed in this group. It would therefore be interesting to test this paradigm for detecting command-following first in this population (asking the patient to count either "yes" or "no") before using it for communication.

Pokorny et al. (2013) tested another auditory P3-based BCI based on tone stream segregation allowing for binary decisions in patients with "MCS" (one VS/UWS with atypical features, 10 MCS, one exit MCS).[3] The patient was presented with two tone streams with infrequently and randomly appearing deviant tones. He was asked to count the number of deviants in one stream in order to elicit a P3 response in the attended stream. Out of the 12 patients included in the study, only five could achieve results above chance level, and none of them achieved performances allowing communication with the system. Response to command could be detected in nine patients after averaging all the responses obtained, although in two of them the response duration was very short (between 30 and 60 ms). It is of interest to note that the paradigm was first developed in healthy controls and had to be adapted to be usable with patients with DOC, reflecting the difficulty of applying a paradigm efficient in non-neurologically impaired subjects to brain-injured subjects. Modifications to the paradigm included: using fewer electrodes; adding a simple paradigm to habituate the patient to the task and to test the presence of a P3 response; using blocks of five consecutive trials with the same target stream instead of a randomized order to decrease the cognitive load; and adding auditorily-presented instructions at the beginning of each run.

Coyle et al. (2015) recently reported the potential use of a motor imagery-based BCI to detect command-following in patients with DOC. This study, which included four MCS patients trained over multiple sessions, highlighted the usefulness of real-time visual and/or auditory feedback to increase alertness and motivation. Limited information was provided regarding the behavioral patterns of these patients, which prevented interpretation in terms of false negatives. This study also reported that musical auditory feedback had a better effect than pink noise or visual feedbacks.

Finally, the usefulness of using hybrid BCIs based on combined brain response has been suggested by Pan and colleagues (2014). In this study, the subject's own face and an unfamiliar face were randomly displayed on the left and right side of a computer screen. The left and right images flickered from appearance to disappearance at different frequencies while the two images also flashed from appearance to disappearance in a random order, eliciting both steady state visually evoked potential (oscillatory electrical responses of neurons in the visual cortex to stimuli flashing at frequencies above 6 Hz) and P3 responses. Four healthy subjects, seven patients with DOC, and one LIS patient were included in the study. All of the healthy subjects, one of the four VS/UWS patients, one of the three MCS patients, and the LIS patient were able to selectively attend to their own or the unfamiliar image (66–100% classification accuracy). Two other patients (one VS/UWS and one MCS) failed to attend the unfamiliar image (50–52% classification accuracy) but achieved significant accuracies for their own image (64–68%). All other patients failed to show any significant response to command. None of the patients with DOC showed response to command at the bedside.

Alternative non-cortically based techniques

Previously presented work has classically focused on systems using sophisticated EEG or fMRI techniques. These may be practical for research and clinical diagnosis but they become challenging in daily use. For this reason, other techniques have also been used and tested in patients with DOC to detect motor-independent response to command at the bedside, such as electromyography (EMG; recording of muscle activity), the measurement of the pupil, and the breathing response.

Bekinschtein et al. studied 10 patients with DOC using EMG (Bekinschtein, Coleman, Niklison, Pickard, & Manes, 2008). Two different commands were

Table 5.1 Studies on paraclinical assessments (i.e., active tasks and brain–computer interfaces) in patients with DOC for assessing response to command and communication.

References	Modality	Task	Targeted (brain) response	Number of patients included
		fMRI and EEG using active tasks		
Owen et al. (2006) & Monti et al. (2010)	fMRI	Playing tennis vs. walking through your house (command-following & communication)	Activation in the supplementary motor area vs. the parahippocampal gyrus	55 (24VS/UWS; 31 MCS)
Bardin et al. (2011)	fMRI	Swimming (command-following & communication)	Activation in the supplementary motor area	6 (3 MCS; 2 exit MCS; 1 LIS)
Monti et al. (2009)	fMRI	Count a target word – neutral (command-following)	Activation in frontoparietal network	1 (MCS)
Naci and Owen (2013)	fMRI	Count a target word – neutral (command-following & communication)	Activation in frontoparietal network	3 (1 VS/UWS; 2 MCS)
Schnakers et al. (2009; 2008b)	EEG	Count a target word – subject's own name (command-following)	P3 response	23 (8VS/UWS; 14 MCS; 1 LIS)
Goldfine et al. (2011b)	EEG	Swimming vs. walking through your house (command-following)	Event-related desynchronization/synchronization in motor areas	3 (1 MCS, 1MCS/exit MCS, 1 LIS)
Cruse et al. (2011; 2012a)	EEG	Squeeze your right hand vs. move your toes (command-following)	Event-related desynchronization/synchronization in motor areas	39 (16 VS/UWS; 23 MCS)
Cruse et al. (2012b)	EEG	Squeeze your right vs. left hand (command-following)	Event-related desynchronization/synchronization in motor areas	1 (VS/UWS)
Chennu et al. (2013)	EEG (20 patients also seen with fMRI active task used in Owen et al. (2006)	Count the number of target words (command-following)	P3 response	21 (9VS/UWS; 12 MCS)

(Continued)

Table 5.1 Continued

References	Modality	Task	Targeted (brain) response	Number of patients included
		Brain–computer interfaces (BCI)		
Lulé et al. (2013)	EEG P3-based BCI	Count a target word (communication)	P3 response	18 (3VS/UWS; 13 MCS; 2 LIS)
Pokorny et al. (2013)	EEG P3-based BCI	Count the number of deviant tones (command-following & communication)	P3 response	12 (1 VS/UWS, 10 MCS, 1 exit MCS)
Coyle et al. (2015)	EEG motor imagery-based BCI	Squeeze your right hand vs. move your toes (command-following)	Event-related desynchronization/ synchronization in motor areas	4 (MCS)
Pan et al. (2014)	EEG hybrid BCI	Count the number of times a target image flashes (command-following)	Steady-state visually evoked response in the occipital area and P3 response	8 (4VS/UWS, 3 MCS, 1 LIS)
		Alternative techniques		
Bekinschtein et al. (2008)	Electromyography	Move your left/right hand (command-following)	Muscular response	10 (8 VS/UWS, 2 MCS)
Habbal et al. (2014)	Electromyography	Move your hands/move your legs/ clench your teeth (command-following)	Muscular response	38 (10 VS/UWS, 28 MCS)
Stoll et al. (2013)	Infrared camera – pupil measurement	Perform an arithmetic problem to select "yes" or "no" response (communication/command-following)	Pupil dilation	12 (7 typical LIS, 4 severely brain-injured LIS with supratentorial brain injury, 1 MCS)
Charland-Verville et al. (2014)	Breathing control	Sniff to end a music sequence (command-following)	Increase in breathing	25 (11 VS/UWS, 14 MCS)

auditorily presented to the patient: "Please try to move your right hand," and "Please try to move your left hand." At the end of the block the instruction was, "Please do not move, stay still." Two auditory phrases were also used as control conditions: "Today is a sunny day," and "It is raining outside today." They reported that one VS/UWS patient and the two MCS patients (one MCS showed response to command at bedside) demonstrated an increased EMG signal specifically linked to the command, suggesting that EMG could be used to objectively detect residual motor responses in this population. In a follow-up study (Habbal et al., 2014), 38 patients with DOC were asked to "Move your hands," "Move your legs," or "Clench your teeth," as compared with a control phrase (i.e., "It is a sunny day"). EMG activity was higher solely for the target command in one patient in a chronic VS/UWS and in three patients in MCS. Out of the 20 patients showing command-following at the bedside, only three could be detected with the system (false negative rate: 85%).

Stoll et al. (2013) investigated the applicability of using pupil dilation, an alternative physiological signal that can be readily and noninvasively measured with robust, inexpensive, and easy-to-use equipment, to communicate with motor-disabled patients and patients with DOC. Pupil dilation has been related to a variety of cognitive functions and is a response that could be used to circumvent the challenges associated with the practical use of traditional BCI approaches. Eleven LIS patients (with or without supratentorial brain injury) and one MCS patient were included in the study. They were asked to answer 10 to 40 questions (26±9), depending on the level of fatigue, using a binary yes/no response. In order to select the right answer, they had to perform an arithmetic problem when the correct response (e.g., "yes") was auditorily presented, and to relax when the incorrect response was presented (e.g., "no"). They reported that three out of seven LIS patients without supratentorial brain injury achieved performances significantly higher than chance when answering yes/no questions using pupil dilation. However, none of the severely brain-injured LIS patients reached significance. Interestingly, Stoll and colleagues also successfully used pupil response to detect command-following in one MCS patient who showed command-following at the bedside but could not communicate, either behaviorally or with the system.

Finally, a recent study used a breathing-based "sniff controller" as an alternative diagnostic tool to evaluate response to command in 25 patients with DOC (Charland-Verville et al., 2014). Patients were instructed to end the presentation of a music sequence by sniffing vigorously. An automated detection of changes in breathing amplitude was used to end the music and hence provide a feedback to the patient. None of the VS/UWS patients showed a sniff-based response to command. However, one out of 14 patients with MCS was able to willfully modulate his breathing pattern to command on 16/19 trials (accuracy 84%). Interestingly, this patient failed to show any other motor response to command. None of the 11 patients showing command-following at the bedside showed a sniff-based response to command (false negative rate: 100%).

Although preliminary results suggest that these tools may provide bedside methods of detecting command-following and communication with the potential to assist the clinician and improve the accuracy of diagnosis, several limitations prevent their use in patients with DOC. Because EMG still requires the preservation of some residual voluntary muscle activity, it could not be used in patients with severe paralysis or chronic spasticity. Also, pupil response can be altered by the use of centrally-acting drugs and restlessness can lead to noninterpretable results for fMRI and EEG. However, future studies should start by using these alternative systems, in conjunction with EEG and/or fMRI, to investigate the integrity of cognitive function in this population.

Guidelines for future research

Current research is focusing on the detection of an oriented response as proof of an ability to be conscious. However, the observed false negative rate remains high with every technique. As the impact of false positive and false negative results is too significant to be disregarded, it is necessary to better understand the exact meaning of the presence or the absence of an expected signal before it will be possible to implement any of these techniques in a clinical setting (Cruse et al., 2013; Goldfine et al., 2013; Pazart, Gabriel, Cretin, & Aubry, 2015).

Indeed, a system that is not sensitive to detecting patients diagnosed as conscious at the bedside could not be reliably used in patients with unclear diagnoses. Similarly, a system that is very sensitive and that detects signs of consciousness in all patients behaviorally diagnosed as conscious, but also in a majority of unconscious patients, would not be specific enough to be reliable for clinicians.

Currently, research on paraclinical assessment tools in patients with DOC will have to overcome several challenges before implementation in clinical settings:

1   **Paradigm complexity**: Brain-injured patients are likely to present arousal fluctuation, fatigue, and limited attention span (Giacino et al., 2002). For this reason, paradigm complexity (stimulus, instructions) and duration are important factors to consider when implementing a system into clinical practice. If the patient shows response to command with the system, communication should be assessed with simple questions since severely brain-damaged patients may have difficulty giving accurate answers to simple yes/no questions (Nakase-Richardson, Yablon, Sherer, Nick, & Evans, 2009).

2   **Sensory deficits**: BCI research in healthy participants seems to suggest better performance with a visual, as compared to auditory or tactile, BCI (Halder et al., 2010; Kubler et al., 2009; Pham et al., 2005). However, current visual BCIs depend on gaze control, which limits their applicability in this population whose severe disabilities can include impaired or nonexistent ocular motor control. Gaze-independent visual BCIs have been proposed in LIS (Lesenfants et al., 2014) but have not yet been evaluated in DOC. Severe deficits, such as cortical deafness, blindness, or oculomotor impairments, also have to be taken into account when working with

brain-damaged patients (Alvarez et al., 2012; Lew et al., 2009; Pogoda et al., 2012; Rowe et al., 2013). The key challenge is therefore to develop reliable systems offering stimuli, instruction, and/or question presentation through multiple modalities. A recent study reporting the applicability of a vibrotactile P3-based tool in LIS patients might enable us to provide systems using a wider range of modalities that take various sensory deficits into account (Lugo et al., 2014). In addition, hybrid BCIs could help improve the sensitivity of the system by combining the use of different brain responses or modalities (Pan et al., 2014), but with an increase in complexity. Future systems should also incorporate a passive evaluation of sensory pathways prior to the active task to help select the more appropriate modality.

3   **Cerebral reorganization/preservation**: Following a brain injury, specific damage in brain areas, together with a certain amount of cerebral reorganization, is likely to occur. This sometimes results in the recruitment of other brain areas during the performance of a given cognitive task, which limits a direct comparison between results observed in patients and in healthy controls (Chennu et al., 2013; Nam, Woo, & Bahn, 2012). Therefore, assessment tools including a range of cognitive abilities supported by spatially-distinct brain regions and indexed by multiple neural signatures are necessary in order to accurately characterize a patient's level of consciousness (Gibson et al., 2014). The inclusion of conscious brain-injured patients could also help researchers interpret the findings in DOC.

4   **Data quality**: Suboptimal data quality due to movement and ocular and respiration artifacts in these challenging populations may also be confounding factors that need to be overcome with the assistance of appropriate statistical analyses that can increase detection of false negatives and positives (Cruse et al., 2013; Goldfine et al., 2013; Goldfine et al., 2011a).

5   **Inter-session variability**: Heterogeneity in achieved performance, correlated or not with the user training, is frequently observed between repetitive assessments in fully conscious participants with the same condition and paradigm. Inter-session variability is not such a big issue in healthy volunteers showing classification accuracy substantially above chance level. However, classification performance in the context of severe brain injury is often close to chance level and a small decrease or increase could potentially be associated with a different diagnostic. Repetitive BCI evaluation must be considered to ensure a reliable diagnosis and to take into account inter-session classification and awareness fluctuation. This would require light, portable, and accessible systems available at the bedside.

6   **Intra-session variability**: Attention and fatigue are difficult to evaluate with noninteracting patients showing arousal/consciousness fluctuation at different times, and these fluctuations could potentially lead to classification performance changes over time and the wrong diagnostic. Trial rejection methods, such as Spatial-Temporal Discriminant Analysis (Zhang et al., 2013) and Step-Wise Linear Discriminant Analysis (Krusienski

et al., 2006), have been proposed to reduce the effect of limited attention and maximize the discriminant information between classes. Extraction of attention measure from the recording during the assessment should also be considered in future developments to better characterize BCI performance changes over time.

7 **Chance level:** The presence of a response to command is generally evaluated with a classification process. Chance level with a confidence interval is used as a threshold to distinguish conscious from unconscious patients. However, several parameters, for example the number of trials and classes, have been shown to influence this threshold (Müller-Putz, Scherer, Brunner, Leeb, & Pfurtscheller, 2008). There is still no consensus defining the most appropriate statistical methods to define significant results, and some results have been controverted following reanalysis of the data (Noirhomme et al., 2014).

8 **Lack of motivation:** The success of active paradigms relies on the patient's willingness to do the task, which might be decreased in case of loss of motivation (Kleih, Nijboer, Halder, & Kubler, 2010; Nijboer et al., 2010) or akinetic mutism (Giacino, 1997; "The permanent vegetative state," 1996). These factors must be considered with care, as we cannot distinguish between a patient lacking motivation to do the task, an unsuccessful patient, and an unconscious patient. One way to increase motivation and control from the patient is to provide a feedback through a BCI system (Coyle et al., 2015; Lulé et al., 2013).

9 **Personalized paradigms:** In the future, researchers and clinicians should start taking into account both the patient's own life experiences and the subjective feelings of their close relatives. Tailoring paradigms to the patient's previous habits may help to increase the sensitivity of these systems (e.g., select familiar actions for motor imagery; Gibson et al., 2013). Interviews with the patient's relatives or caregivers can help select specific stimuli "known" to induce some signs of responsiveness at the bedside, such as a given surname, a familiar voice, or a specific song. Even if these responses are not always clinically reproducible or objective, a detectable response may be objectified by one of the techniques presented above (Pazart et al., 2015).

10 **Ethical implications:** Finally, the implementation of paraclinical tools for detection of command-following and communication in clinical settings will have to be wisely managed in order to define clear guidelines for clinicians in terms of interpretation and use of the findings in their discussions with families as well as the implications for care (i.e., pain management) and end-of-life decisions (see Chapter 7).

Altogether, paraclinical assessments may offer many possibilities for patients with DOC and could have a major impact on care and quality of life in this population. However, further work must be done before these assessments can be used as a supplemental tool to the current behavioral "gold standard" for assessment of consciousness. An extensive collaborative project between researchers, including data sharing to enable comparison between paradigms, analyses, and patients' demographics and clinical data, is also needed to efficiently address the issues highlighted above. In addition, studies will need to focus not only on the decrease of false negatives, but also on the decrease of false positives in order to develop reliable tools for clinicians.

In the future, BCIs could help us detect cognitive impairment at an early stage, using a binary communication code (Schnakers et al., 2008a) with such systems (Müller-Putz, Pokorny, Klobassa, & Horki, 2013), and they could help us to guide rehabilitation programs accordingly.

BCIs could also be used for motor rehabilitation in patients with DOC, as previous literature has suggested that motor imagery training could induce a modification of cortical activity in healthy volunteers and stroke patients (Dickstein et al., 2014; Page, Szaflarski, Eliassen, Pan, & Cramer, 2009; Pichiorri et al., 2011; Santos-Couto-Paz, Teixeira-Salmela, & Tierra-Criollo, 2013; for a review, see Teo & Chew, 2014) and help in the recovery of motor function of paralyzed limbs (Jackson, Lafleur, Malouin, Richards, & Doyon, 2001; Oostra, Vereecke, Jones, Vanderstraeten, & Vingerhoets, 2012; Page, Levine, & Leonard, 2007; Prasad, Herman, Coyle, McDonough, & Crosbie, 2010; Sacco et al., 2011).

Finally, it is important to note that, in order to use any of the paradigms presented above, the patient will need to be able to understand the task requirements. Therefore we need to be cautious, as these systems will not be sensitive to detect patients suffering from language impairments (Majerus, Bruno, Schnakers, Giacino, & Laureys, 2009). In these cases, language-independent paradigms will be needed (for a review, see Boly & Seth, 2012; e.g., Casali et al., 2013; Faugeras et al., 2011; King et al., 2013; Malinowska et al., 2013; Phillips et al., 2011).

Conclusion

In this chapter, we provided a state-of-the-art on the development of paraclinical tools for diagnosis of patients with DOC. We highlighted the main challenges that need to be overcome before these systems could be used for care management and rehabilitation strategies in this population. Despite the increased interest and medialization of the positive findings, results obtained in patients with DOC will need to be interpreted with caution. Results from these studies suggest that the likelihood that a covertly aware patient might go undetected (i.e., the false negative rate) is likely to vary significantly across different paradigms and remains generally high (Chatelle et al., 2015). In the future, the suitability of different methods (modalities, brain response) for single patients will need to be assessed on a case-by-case basis in order to increase the reliability of the system. While some patients have been shown to consistently perform sensorimotor response to command using EEG, others were able to perform mental imagery in the fMRI (Gibson et al., 2014). Hence, none of these tests applied alone can currently be used to interpret negative results without combining findings from multiple testing methods to mitigate against the level of uncertainty. Likewise, positive findings should not be taken as clear evidence of consciousness but should rather be used as an opportunity to discuss clinical findings and, in case of discordance, to further explore reasons for the discrepancy.

Acknowledgments

This study was supported by the Belgian American Educational Foundation (BAEF), the Fédération Wallonie Bruxelles International (WBI), the Massachusetts General Hospital Department of Neurology and Division of Neurocritical Care and Emergency Neurology, the French Speaking Community Concerted Research Action (ARC), the James McDonnell Foundation, and the Léon Frédéricq Foundation.

Notes

1 **Camille Chatelle** is a postdoctoral research fellow at the Neurorehabilitation Lab at the Spaulding Rehabilitation Hospital, Harvard Medical School. She is also working as a postdoctoral researcher at the Laboratory for NeuroImaging of Coma and Consciousness at Massachusetts General Hospital, Harvard Medical School.
2 **Damien Lesenfants** is a postdoctoral research associate in Engineering in the Braingate project (Brown University, Massachusetts General Hospital, Stanford University, and Providence VA Medical Center) and participates actively in the research of the Coma Science Group, University of Liège, Liège, Belgium.
3 Based on CRS-R data obtained from Pokorny et al. (2013). Note that subscores were missing for four patients, which prevented interpretation of false negatives.

References

Alvarez, T. L., Kim, E. H., Vicci, V. R., Dhar, S. K., Biswal, B. B., & Barrett, A. M. (2012). Concurrent vision dysfunctions in convergence insufficiency with traumatic brain injury. *Optom Vis Sci, 89*(12), 1740–1751.

Bai, O., Lin, P., Vorbach, S., Floeter, M. K., Hattori, N., & Hallett, M. (2008). A high performance sensorimotor beta rhythm-based brain-computer interface associated with human natural motor behavior. *J Neural Eng, 5*(1), 24–35.

Bardin, J. C., Fins, J. J., Katz, D. I., Hersh, J., Heier, L. A., Tabelow, K., . . . Voss, H. U. (2011). Dissociations between behavioural and functional magnetic resonance imaging-based evaluations of cognitive function after brain injury. *Brain, 134*(Pt 3), 769–782.

Bekinschtein, T. A., Coleman, M. R., Niklison, J., 3rd, Pickard, J. D., & Manes, F. F. (2008). Can electromyography objectively detect voluntary movement in disorders of consciousness? *J Neurol Neurosurg Psychiatry, 79*(7), 826–828.

Birbaumer, N. (2006). Breaking the silence: brain-computer interfaces (BCI) for communication and motor control. *Psychophysiology, 43*(6), 517–532.

Boly, M., & Seth, A. K. (2012). Modes and models in disorders of consciousness science. *Arch Ital Biol, 150*(2–3), 172–184.

Casali, A. G., Gosseries, O., Rosanova, M., Boly, M., Sarasso, S., Casali, K. R., . . . Massimini, M. (2013). A theoretically based index of consciousness independent of sensory processing and behavior. *Sci Transl Med, 5*(198), 198ra105.

Charland-Verville, V., Lesenfants, D., Sela, L., Noirhomme, Q., Ziegler, E., Chatelle, C., . . . Laureys, S. (2014). Detection of response to command using voluntary control of breathing in disorders of consciousness. *Front Hum Neurosci, 8*, 1020.

Chatelle, C., Chennu, S., Noirhomme, Q., Cruse, D., Owen, A. M., & Laureys, S. (2012). Brain-computer interfacing in disorders of consciousness. *Brain Inj, 26*(12), 1510–1522.

Chatelle, C., Lesenfants, D., Guller, Y., Laureys, S., & Noirhomme, Q. (2015). Brain-computer interface for assessing consciousness in severely brain-injured patients. In A. Rossetti & S. Laureys (Eds.), *Clinical Neurophysiology in Disorders of Consciousness* (pp. 133–148). Wien: Springer.

Chennu, S., Finoia, P., Kamau, E., Monti, M. M., Allanson, J., Pickard, J. D., . . . Bekinschtein, T. A. (2013). Dissociable endogenous and exogenous attention in disorders of consciousness. *Neuroimage Clin, 3*, 450–461.

Citi, L., Poli, R., Cinel, C., & Sepulveda, F. (2008). P300-based BCI mouse with genetically-optimized analogue control. *IEEE Trans Neural Syst Rehabil Eng, 16*(1), 51–61.

Combaz, A., Chatelle, C., Robben, A., Vanhoof, G., Goeleven, A., Thijs, V., . . . Laureys, S. (2013). A comparison of two spelling brain-computer interfaces based on visual P3 and SSVEP in locked-in syndrome. *PLoS One, 8*(9), e73691.

Coyle, D., Stow, J., McCreadie, K., McElligott, J., & Carroll, A. (2015). Sensorimotor modulation assessment and brain-computer interface training in disorders of consciousness. *Arch Phys Med Rehabil, 96*(3 Suppl), S62–70.

Cruse, D., Chennu, S., Chatelle, C., Bekinschtein, T., Fernández-Espejo, D., Junqué, C., . . . and Owen, A. (2011). Bedside detection of awareness in the vegetative state. *The Lancet, 378*(9809), 2088–2094.

Cruse, D., Chennu, S., Chatelle, C., Bekinschtein, T. A., Fernández-Espejo, D., Pickard, J. D., . . . Owen, A. M. (2013). Reanalysis of "Bedside detection of awareness in the vegetative state: a cohort study" – Authors' reply. *Lancet, 381*(9863), 291–292.

Cruse, D., Chennu, S., Chatelle, C., Fernández-Espejo, D., Bekinschtein, T. A., Pickard, J., . . . Owen, A. M. (2012a). The relationship between aetiology and covert cognition in the minimally-conscious state. *Neurology, 78*(11), 816–822.

Cruse, D., Chennu, S., Fernández-Espejo, D., Payne, W. L., Young, G. B., & Owen, A. M. (2012b). Detecting awareness in the vegetative state: electroencephalographic evidence for attempted movements to command. *PLoS One, 7*(11), e49933.

Dickstein, R., Levy, S., Shefi, S., Holtzman, S., Peleg, S., & Vatine, J. J. (2014). Motor imagery group practice for gait rehabilitation in individuals with post-stroke hemiparesis: a pilot study. *NeuroRehabilitation, 34*(2), 267–276.

Faugeras, F., Rohaut, B., Weiss, N., Bekinschtein, T. A., Galanaud, D., Puybasset, L., . . . Naccache, L. (2011). Probing consciousness with event-related potentials in the vegetative state. *Neurology, 77*(3), 264–268.

Fernández-Espejo, D., & Owen, A. M. (2013). Detecting awareness after severe brain injury. *Nat Rev Neurosci, 14*(11), 801–809.

Giacino, J., Ashwal, S., Childs, N., Cranford, R., Jennett, B., Katz, D., . . . Zafonte, R. (2002). The minimally conscious state: definition and diagnostic criteria. *Neurology, 58*(3), 349–353.

Giacino, J. T. (1997). Disorders of consciousness: differential diagnosis and neuropathologic features. *Semin Neurol, 17*(2), 105–111.

Gibson, R. M., Chennu, S., Owen, A. M., & Cruse, D. (2013). Complexity and familiarity enhance single-trial detectability of imagined movements with electroencephalography. *Clin Neurophysiol, 125*(8), 1556–1567.

Gibson, R. M., Fernández-Espejo, D., Gonzalez-Lara, L. E., Kwan, B. Y., Lee, D. H., Owen, A. M., & Cruse, D. (2014). Multiple tasks and neuroimaging modalities increase the likelihood of detecting covert awareness in patients with disorders of consciousness. *Front Hum Neurosci, 8*, 950.

Goldfine, A. M., Bardin, J. C., Noirhomme, Q., Fins, J. J., Schiff, N. D., & Victor, J. D. (2013). Reanalysis of "Bedside detection of awareness in the vegetative state: a cohort study." *The Lancet, 381*(9863), 289–291.

Goldfine, A. M., Victor, J. D., Conte, M. M., Bardin, J. C., & Schiff, N. D. (2011a). Determination of awareness in patients with severe brain injury using EEG power spectral analysis. *Clin Neurophysiol, 122*(11), 2157–2168.

Habbal, D., Gosseries, O., Noirhomme, Q., Renaux, J., Lesenfants, D., Bekinschtein, T. A., . . . Schnakers, C. (2014). Volitional electromyographic responses in disorders of consciousness. *Brain Inj, 28*(9), 1171–1179.

Halder, S., Rea, M., Andreoni, R., Nijboer, F., Hammer, E. M., Kleih, S. C., . . . Kubler, A. (2010). An auditory oddball brain-computer interface for binary choices. *Clin Neurophysiol, 121*(4), 516–523.

Hochberg, L. R., Bacher, D., Jarosiewicz, B., Masse, N. Y., Simeral, J. D., Vogel, J., . . . Donoghue, J. P. (2012). Reach and grasp by people with tetraplegia using a neurally controlled robotic arm. *Nature, 485*(7398), 372–375.

Hochberg, L. R., Serruya, M. D., Friehs, G. M., Mukand, J. A., Saleh, M., Caplan, A. H., . . . Donoghue, J. P. (2006). Neuronal ensemble control of prosthetic devices by a human with tetraplegia. *Nature, 442*(7099), 164–171.

Jackson, P. L., Lafleur, M. F., Malouin, F., Richards, C., & Doyon, J. (2001). Potential role of mental practice using motor imagery in neurologic rehabilitation. *Arch Phys Med Rehabil, 82*(8), 1133–1141.

King, J. R., Sitt, J. D., Faugeras, F., Rohaut, B., El Karoui, I., Cohen, L., . . . Dehaene, S. (2013). Information sharing in the brain indexes consciousness in noncommunicative patients. *Curr Biol, 23*(19), 1914–1919.

Kleih, S. C., Nijboer, F., Halder, S., & Kubler, A. (2010). Motivation modulates the P300 amplitude during brain-computer interface use. *Clin Neurophysiol, 121*(7), 1023–1031.

Krusienski, D. J., Sellers, E. W., Cabestaing, F., Bayoudh, S., McFarland, D. J., Vaughan, T. M., & Wolpaw, J. R. (2006). A comparison of classification techniques for the P300 Speller. *J Neural Eng, 3*(4), 299–305.

Kubler, A., & Birbaumer, N. (2008). Brain-computer interfaces and communication in paralysis: extinction of goal directed thinking in completely paralysed patients? *Clin Neurophysiol, 119*(11), 2658–2666.

Kubler, A., Furdea, A., Halder, S., Hammer, E. M., Nijboer, F., & Kotchoubey, B. (2009). A brain-computer interface controlled auditory event-related potential (p300) spelling system for locked-in patients. *Ann N Y Acad Sci, 1157*, 90–100.

Kubler, A., Mushahwar, V. K., Hochberg, L. R., & Donoghue, J. P. (2006). BCI Meeting 2005 – workshop on clinical issues and applications. *IEEE Trans Neural Syst Rehabil Eng, 14*(2), 131–134.

Kubler, A., Nijboer, F., Mellinger, J., Vaughan, T. M., Pawelzik, H., Schalk, G., . . . Wolpaw, J. R. (2005). Patients with ALS can use sensorimotor rhythms to operate a brain-computer interface. *Neurology, 64*(10), 1775–1777.

Laureys, S., Pellas, F., Van Eeckhout, P., Ghorbel, S., Schnakers, C., Perrin, F., . . . Goldman, S. (2005). The locked-in syndrome: what is it like to be conscious but paralyzed and voiceless? *Prog Brain Res, 150*, 495–511.

Lee, J. H., Ryu, J., Jolesz, F. A., Cho, Z. H., & Yoo, S. S. (2009). Brain-machine interface via real-time fMRI: preliminary study on thought-controlled robotic arm. *Neurosci Lett, 450*(1), 1–6.

Lesenfants, D., Habbal, D., Lugo, Z., Lebeau, M., Horki, P., Amico, E., . . . Noirhomme, Q. (2014). An independent SSVEP-based brain-computer interface in locked-in syndrome. *J Neural Eng, 11*(3), 035002.

Lew, H. L., Garvert, D. W., Pogoda, T. K., Hsu, P. T., Devine, J. M., White, D. K., . . . Goodrich, G. L. (2009). Auditory and visual impairments in patients with blast-related traumatic brain injury: effect of dual sensory impairment on Functional Independence Measure. *J Rehabil Res Dev, 46*(6), 819–826.

Lugo, Z. R., Rodriguez, J., Lechner, A., Ortner, R., Gantner, I. S., Laureys, S., . . . Guger, C. (2014). A vibrotactile p300-based brain-computer interface for consciousness detection and communication. *Clin EEG Neurosci, 45*(1), 14–21.

Lulé, D., Noirhomme, Q., Kleih, S. C., Chatelle, C., Halder, S., Demertzi, A., . . . Laureys, S. (2013). Probing command following in patients with disorders of consciousness using a brain-computer interface. *Clin Neurophysiol, 124*(1), 101–106.

Majerus, S., Bruno, M. A., Schnakers, C., Giacino, J. T., & Laureys, S. (2009). The problem of aphasia in the assessment of consciousness in brain-damaged patients. *Prog Brain Res, 177,* 49–61.

Malinowska, U., Chatelle, C., Bruno, M. A., Noirhomme, Q., Laureys, S., & Durka, P. J. (2013). Electroencephalographic profiles for differentiation of disorders of consciousness. *Biomed Eng Online, 12*(1), 109.

Monti, M. M., Coleman, M. R., & Owen, A. M. (2009). Executive functions in the absence of behavior: functional imaging of the minimally conscious state. *Prog Brain Res, 177,* 249–260.

Monti, M. M., Vanhaudenhuyse, A., Coleman, M. R., Boly, M., Pickard, J. D., Tshibanda, L., . . . Laureys, S. (2010). Willful modulation of brain activity in disorders of consciousness. *N Engl J Med, 362*(7), 579–589.

Mugler, E. M., Ruf, C. A., Halder, S., Bensch, M., & Kler, A. (2010). Design and implementation of a P300-based brain-computer interface for controlling an internet browser. *IEEE Trans Neural Syst Rehabil Eng, 18*(6), 599–609.

Müller-Putz, G., Scherer, R., Brunner, C., Leeb, R., & Pfurtscheller, G. (2008). Better than random? A closer look on BCI results. *International Journal of Bioelectromagnetism, 10*(1), 52–55.

Müller-Putz, G. R., Pokorny, C., Klobassa, D. S., & Horki, P. (2013). A single-switch BCI based on passive and imagined movements: toward restoring communication in minimally conscious patients. *International Journal of Neural Systems, 23*(2), 1250037.

Naci, L., & Owen, A. M. (2013). Making every word count for nonresponsive patients. *JAMA Neurol, 70*(10), 1235–1241.

Nakase-Richardson, R., Yablon, S. A., Sherer, M., Nick, T. G., & Evans, C. C. (2009). Emergence from minimally conscious state: insights from evaluation of posttraumatic confusion. *Neurology, 73*(14), 1120–1126.

Nam, C. S., Woo, J., & Bahn, S. (2012). Severe motor disability affects functional cortical integration in the context of brain-computer interface (BCI) use. *Ergonomics, 55*(5), 581–591.

Neuper, C., Müller-Putz, G. R., Kubler, A., Birbaumer, N., & Pfurtscheller, G. (2003). Clinical application of an EEG-based brain-computer interface: a case study in a patient with severe motor impairment. *Clin Neurophysiol, 114*(3), 399–409.

Neuper, C., Scherer, R., Reiner, M., & Pfurtscheller, G. (2005). Imagery of motor actions: differential effects of kinesthetic and visual-motor mode of imagery in single-trial EEG. *Brain Res Cogn Brain Res, 25*(3), 668–677.

Nijboer, F., Birbaumer, N., & Kubler, A. (2010). The influence of psychological state and motivation on brain-computer interface performance in patients with amyotrophic lateral sclerosis – a longitudinal study. *Front Neurosci, 4,* 55.

Noirhomme, Q., Lesenfants, D., Gomez, F., Soddu, A., Schrouff, J., Garraux, G., . . . Laureys, S. (2014). Biased binomial assessment of cross-validated estimation of classification accuracies illustrated in diagnosis predictions. *Neuroimage Clin, 4*, 687–694.

Oostra, K. M., Vereecke, A., Jones, K., Vanderstraeten, G., & Vingerhoets, G. (2012). Motor imagery ability in patients with traumatic brain injury. *Arch Phys Med Rehabil, 93*(5), 828–833.

Owen, A. M., Coleman, M. R., Boly, M., Davis, M. H., Laureys, S., & Pickard, J. D. (2006). Detecting awareness in the vegetative state. *Science, 313*(5792), 1402.

Page, S. J., Levine, P., & Leonard, A. (2007). Mental practice in chronic stroke: results of a randomized, placebo-controlled trial. *Stroke, 38*(4), 1293–1297.

Page, S. J., Szaflarski, J. P., Eliassen, J. C., Pan, H., & Cramer, S. C. (2009). Cortical plasticity following motor skill learning during mental practice in stroke. *Neurorehabil Neural Repair, 23*(4), 382–388.

Pan, J., Xie, Q., He, Y., Wang, F., Di, H., Laureys, S., . . . Li, Y. (2014). Detecting awareness in patients with disorders of consciousness using a hybrid brain-computer interface. *J Neural Eng, 11*(5), 056007.

Pazart, L., Gabriel, D., Cretin, E., & Aubry, R. (2015). Neuroimaging for detecting covert awareness in patients with disorders of consciousness: reinforce the place of clinical feeling! *Front Hum Neurosci, 9*, 78.

The permanent vegetative state. (1996). Review by a working group convened by the Royal College of Physicians and endorsed by the Conference of Medical Royal Colleges and their faculties of the United Kingdom. *J R Coll Physicians Lond, 30*(2), 119–121.

Pfurtscheller, G., & Lopes da Silva, F. H. (1999). Event-related EEG/MEG synchronization and desynchronization: basic principles. *Clin Neurophysiol, 110*(11), 1842–1857.

Pfurtscheller, G., Neuper, C., Flotzinger, D., & Pregenzer, M. (1997). EEG-based discrimination between imagination of right and left hand movement. *Electroencephalogr Clin Neurophysiol, 103*(6), 642–651.

Pham, M., Hinterberger, T., Neumann, N., Kubler, A., Hofmayer, N., Grether, A., . . . Birbaumer, N. (2005). An auditory brain-computer interface based on the self-regulation of slow cortical potentials. *Neurorehabil Neural Repair, 19*(3), 206–218.

Phillips, C. L., Bruno, M. A., Maquet, P., Boly, M., Noirhomme, Q., Schnakers, C., . . . Laureys, S. (2011). "Relevance vector machine" consciousness classifier applied to cerebral metabolism of vegetative and locked-in patients. *Neuroimage, 56*(2), 797–808.

Piccione, F., Giorgi, F., Tonin, P., Priftis, K., Giove, S., Silvoni, S., . . . Beverina, F. (2006). P300-based brain computer interface: reliability and performance in healthy and paralysed participants. *Clin Neurophysiol, 117*(3), 531–537.

Pichiorri, F., De Vico Fallani, F., Cincotti, F., Babiloni, F., Molinari, M., Kleih, S. C., . . . Mattia, D. (2011). Sensorimotor rhythm-based brain-computer interface training: the impact on motor cortical responsiveness. *J Neural Eng, 8*(2), 025020.

Pogoda, T. K., Hendricks, A. M., Iverson, K. M., Stolzmann, K. L., Krengel, M. H., Baker, E., . . . Lew, H. L. (2012). Multisensory impairment reported by veterans with and without mild traumatic brain injury history. *J Rehabil Res Dev, 49*(7), 971–984.

Pokorny, C., Klobassa, D. S., Pichler, G., Erlbeck, H., Real, R. G., Kubler, A., . . . Muller-Putz, G. R. (2013). The auditory P300-based single-switch brain-computer interface: paradigm transition from healthy subjects to minimally conscious patients. *Artif Intell Med, 59*(2), 81–90.

Polich, J. (2007). Updating P300: an integrative theory of P3a and P3b. *Clin Neurophysiol, 118*(10), 2128–2148.

Prasad, G., Herman, P., Coyle, D., McDonough, S., & Crosbie, J. (2010). Applying a brain-computer interface to support motor imagery practice in people with stroke for upper limb recovery: a feasibility study. *J Neuroeng Rehabil, 7*, 60.

Risetti, M., Formisano, R., Toppi, J., Quitadamo, L. R., Bianchi, L., Astolfi, L., . . . Mattia, D. (2013). On ERPs detection in disorders of consciousness rehabilitation. *Front Hum Neurosci, 7*, 775.

Rowe, F. J., Wright, D., Brand, D., Jackson, C., Harrison, S., Maan, T., . . . Freeman, C. (2013). A prospective profile of visual field loss following stroke: prevalence, type, rehabilitation, and outcome. *Biomed Res Int, 2013*, 719096.

Sacco, K., Cauda, F., D'Agata, F., Duca, S., Zettin, M., Virgilio, R., . . . Geminiani, G. (2011). A combined robotic and cognitive training for locomotor rehabilitation: evidences of cerebral functional reorganization in two chronic traumatic brain injured patients. *Front Hum Neurosci, 5*, 146.

Santos-Couto-Paz, C. C., Teixeira-Salmela, L. F., & Tierra-Criollo, C. J. (2013). The addition of functional task-oriented mental practice to conventional physical therapy improves motor skills in daily functions after stroke. *Braz J Phys Ther, 17*(6), 564–571.

Schnakers, C., Majerus, S., Goldman, S., Boly, M., Van Eeckhout, P., Gay, S., . . . Laureys, S. (2008a). Cognitive function in the locked-in syndrome. *J Neurol, 255*(3), 323–330.

Schnakers, C., Perrin, F., Schabus, M., Hustinx, R., Majerus, S., Moonen, G., . . . Laureys, S. (2009). Detecting consciousness in a total locked-in syndrome: an active event-related paradigm. *Neurocase, 4*, 1–7.

Schnakers, C., Perrin, F., Schabus, M., Majerus, S., Ledoux, D., Damas, P., . . . Laureys, S. (2008b). Voluntary brain processing in disorders of consciousness. *Neurology, 71*, 1614–1620.

Sellers, E. W., & Donchin, E. (2006). A P300-based brain-computer interface: initial tests by ALS patients. *Clin Neurophysiol, 117*(3), 538–548.

Sellers, E. W., Kubler, A., & Donchin, E. (2006). Brain-computer interface research at the University of South Florida Cognitive Psychophysiology Laboratory: the P300 Speller. *IEEE Trans Neural Syst Rehabil Eng, 14*(2), 221–224.

Sellers, E. W., Vaughan, T. M., & Wolpaw, J. R. (2010). A brain-computer interface for long-term independent home use. *Amyotroph Lateral Scler, 11*(5), 449–455.

Stoll, J., Chatelle, C., Carter, O., Koch, C., Laureys, S., & Einhauser, W. (2013). Pupil responses allow communication in locked-in syndrome patients. *Curr Biol, 23*(15), R647–648.

Teo, W. P., & Chew, E. (2014). Is motor-imagery brain-computer interface feasible in stroke rehabilitation? A narrative review. *PM R, 6*(8), 723–728.

Wolpaw, J. R., Birbaumer, N., McFarland, D. J., Pfurtscheller, G., & Vaughan, T. M. (2002). Brain-computer interfaces for communication and control. *Clin Neurophysiol, 113*(6), 767–791.

Yoo, S. S., Fairneny, T., Chen, N. K., Choo, S. E., Panych, L. P., Park, H., . . . Jolesz, F. A. (2004). Brain-computer interface using fMRI: spatial navigation by thoughts. *Neuroreport, 15*(10), 1591–1595.

Zhang, Y., Zhou, G., Zhao, Q., Jin, J., Wang, X., & Cichocki, A. (2013). Spatial-temporal discriminant analysis for ERP-based brain-computer interface. *IEEE Trans Neural Syst Rehabil Eng, 21*(2), 233–243.

6 Brain-computer interface (BCI) communication in the locked-in

A tool for differential diagnosis

Ujwal Chaudhary,[1] *Francesco Piccione,*[2] *and Niels Birbaumer*[3]

Abbreviations

AAC	augmentative and alternative communication
ALS	amyotrophic lateral sclerosis
BCI	brain-computer interface
BOLD	blood oxygen level-dependent
CLIS	complete locked-in syndrome
CR	conditioned reaction
CS	conditioned stimulus
ECoG	electrocorticography
EEG	electroencephalography
fMRI	functional magnetic resonance imaging
LFP	local field potential
LIS	locked-in state
MCS	minimally conscious state
MEG	magnetoencephalography
NIRS	near-infrared spectroscopy
PNS	peripheral nerve stimulation
rt-fMRI	real time-functional magnetic resonance imaging
SCP	slow cortical potential
SMR	sensorimotor rhythm
SWS	slow wave sleep
TMS	transcranial magnetic stimulation
US	unconditioned stimulus
VS/UWS	vegetative state/unresponsive wakefulness syndrome

Introduction

Several neurological diseases that destroy the human body's motor functions exist, such as amyotrophic lateral sclerosis (ALS), stroke, muscular dystrophy, high spinal cord injury, and chronic Guillain-Barré Syndrome. The patients suffering from such conditions are said to be in the "locked-in" syndrome (LIS) because they become partially or completely paralyzed and have residual voluntary control over only a few muscles, such as eye movement, eye blinks, or lip twitches. These patients are therefore not in an altered state of consciousness, but they are at high risk of being misdiagnosed as being in a VS/UWS or MCS. The fact that they are capable of processing pain but unable to show it at the bedside (physically or verbally) makes this condition a real challenge for clinicians. To help these patients to communicate, a reliable external pathway must be created to bypass the disrupted efferent pathway such that communication between the brain of the patient and an external device/instrument is possible. Such an interface, which uses brain signals to drive external devices without participation of the spinal and peripheral motor system, is called a brain-computer interface (BCI). Thus BCI aims, among other applications, at establishing a non-muscular communication pathway between the brain and external electronic or mechanical devices. This chapter describes BCI's role in providing a communication tool for patients in LIS. We will particularly focus on the challenge of patients in the complete LIS from ALS, although this can apply to other varieties of LIS as well.

ALS is a progressive motor neuron disease of unknown etiology resulting eventually in a complete destruction of the peripheral and central motor system (Figure 6.1) affecting sensory or cognitive functions to a minor degree (Norris, 1992). Clinical, pathological, and genetic advances indicate heterogeneity in phenotype, pathological substrate, and genetic predisposition, suggesting that ALS should be considered a syndrome rather than a single disease entity (Beleza-Meireles & Al-Chalabi, 2009; Deng, et al., 2010). The course is unalterably progressive. The clinical presentation and progression of ALS vary considerably, and over 60% of patients die within three years after diagnosis if not artificially respirated. Of the remaining patients, up to 10% survive for more than eight years (Kiernan, et al., 2011). However, these types of statistics on survival are highly questionable and based on heterogeneous data acquisition with unknown medical and social contexts determining these numbers.

ALS is familial in 5% of cases, and the clinical phenotype of familial ALS is similar to that of the sporadic form of the disease. At least 15 genes have been associated with the various types of familial ALS, and variants in these genes account for 30% of these cases (Deng, et al., 2010). Sporadic ALS is considered to be a complex disease, in which genetic and environmental factors combine to increase the risk of developing the condition (Deng, et al., 2010). Disease phenotype is often classified by the site of onset, which is usually asymmetrical. The majority (65%) of patients present with limb symptoms, while 30% present with symptoms of bulbar dysfunction in the form of dysarthria or dysphagia. Five percent of patients have respiratory-onset disease (Logroscino, et al., 2010). It is widely believed that neurodegeneration, whether in the motor cortex or in the lower motor neurons (LMN), begins long before the onset of symptomatic weakness (Wohlfart & Wohlfart, 1935; Swash and Ingram, 1988). However, studies of LMN function suggest that both in sporadic ALS (de Carvalho & Swash, 2006) and in familial and juvenile ALS (Aggarwal & Nicholson, 2002)

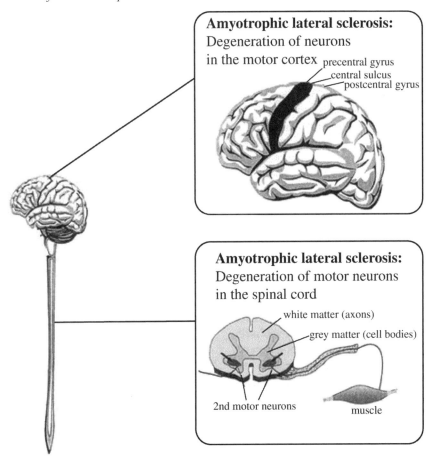

Figure 6.1 Paralysis in amyotrophic lateral sclerosis is caused by degeneration of the first and second motor neurons in the spinal cord and neurons in the motor cortex. (Figure modified and adapted from Kübler et al., 2001.)

weakness is detectable only several months after the commencement of progressive LMN dysfunction. Extraocular and sphincter muscles are characteristically spared in patients with ALS, at least until late in the disease (Eisen, Kim & Pant, 1992), although subtle changes in eye movements have been reported (Donaghy, et al., 2009; Donaghy, et al., 2010).

There is no treatment available; patients have to decide whether to accept artificial respiration and feeding for the rest of their lives after the disease destroys respiratory and bulbar functions or to die of respiratory or related problems. If they opt for life and accept artificial respiration, the disease progresses until the patient loses control of the last muscular response, which is usually the eye muscle or the external sphincter. The resulting condition is called complete locked-in syndrome (CLIS) (Bauer, et al., 1979). CLIS condition consists of virtually total immobility, including all eye movements, combined with preserved consciousness. If there is total immobility except for vertical eye movement and blinking, combined with preserved consciousness, then the patient is said to be in locked-in syndrome (LIS) (Bauer et al., 1979). Almost all people with ALS experience a speech disorder as the disease progresses. Initial symptoms typically do not interfere with speech intelligibility and may be limited to a reduction in spelling rate, a change in phonatory (voice) quality, or imprecise articulation. At some point in the disease progression, 80 to 95% of patients with ALS become unable to meet their daily communication needs using natural speech. Later, most become unable to speak at all (Ball, Beukelman & Bardach, 2007). For these patients, communication support involves a range of augmentative and alternative communication (AAC) strategies involving low- and high-technology (speech-generating devices) options (Beukelman & Mirenda, 2005). Clinical decision-making related to communication is quite complex as screening, referral, assessment, acquisition of technology, and training must occur in a timely manner so that, when residual speech is no longer effective, AAC strategies are in place to support communication related to personal care, medical care, social interaction, community involvement, and perhaps employment. Hence there is a need for an assistive technology to help ALS patients in LIS or CLIS to communicate needs and feelings to their family members/caregivers.

Brain-computer interface

Brain-computer interface (BCI) technology has generated considerable research interest for patients with LIS such as those in the late stages of ALS. BCIs permit action through brain signals such as spike trains from single neurons (Velliste et al., 2008; Riehle & Vaadia, 2005), extracellular local field potentials (LFPs) (Lebedev & Nicolelis, 2006), electrocorticograms (ECoG) (Felton, Wilson, Williams, & Garell, 2007), electroencephalogram (EEG) oscillations (Birbaumer & Cohen, 2007), event-related brain potentials (ERPs) (Nijboer et al., 2008), real time-functional magnetic resonance imaging (rt-fMRI) (Caria et al., 2007), and near-infrared spectroscopy (NIRS) (Sitaram et al., 2007a, 2007b; Gallegos Ayala et al., 2014). In most BCIs, the user's brain activity is acquired via amplifiers, filtered, and decoded using an online classification algorithm. In turn, this output is fed back to users, which allows them to modulate their brain activity. The feedback may consist of: sensory stimuli such as visual (Caria et al., 2007), auditory (Nijboer, Furdea, Gunst, et al., 2008), or vibrotactile stimuli varying proportionally to the classified brain activity; a discrete reward for a particular brain response: a verbal response (such as "yes" or "no"); the movements of a prosthesis or wheelchair; or direct electrical stimulation of muscles or brain. Thus, feedback of the consequences of the brain activity carried out to control the device is likely an essential part of a successful BCI, and it is usually called neurofeedback.

BCI research includes invasive (implantable electrodes on or in the neocortex such as ECoG) and noninvasive means, including EEG, magnetoencephalography (MEG), functional magnetic resonance imaging (fMRI), and NIRS to record brain activity for conveying the user's intent to devices such as simple word-processing programs. Noninvasive methods have been utilized more extensively than invasive methods for people with disabilities (such as those with ALS) (Birbaumer & Cohen 2007; Birbaumer, Murguialday & Cohen, 2008). While those with ALS and other conditions who are in a LIS have motivated research in this area, very few systems have been consistently successful with this population.

Invasive BCIs for communication

The population codes of neural cell assemblies, represented in the firing patterns of its single cells, constitute the substrate for behaviorally relevant information. Whether it is the spiking of cells or the synaptically generated local LFP that holds the key for encoding this information is debatable and probably varies with the behavioral or cognitive demands of the particular assembly (see Abeles, 1991). Regardless, a BCI using the population codes of behaviorally relevant assemblies contains the largest degrees of freedom if the relevant cell assemblies are included and recorded with the implanted electrode array. Kennedy, Kirby, Moore, King, and Mallory (2004) published several single cases with ALS in different stages (none either LIS or CLIS), with a cortically implanted glass microelectrode filled with a neurotrophic growth factor. The axon of the cell targeted by the electrode grows into it and allows recording of the spike activity. Some of the patients learned to spell using the spike activity, mainly by turning it on and off in a "yes" or "no" fashion, but it must be noted that none of the patient were in CLIS. Brunner, Graimann, Huggins, Levine, and Pfurtscheller (2005), Graimann, Huggins, Levine, and Pfurtscheller (2004), and Pfurtscheller, Mueller, Pfurtscheller, Gerner, and Rupp (2003) implanted subdural electrodes in presurgical epileptic patients and demonstrated that control of sensorimotor rhythm (SMR) synchronization and desynchronization can be achieved in one to several sessions. A series of BCI studies on human patients with subdurally or epidurally implanted macroelectrodes recording ECoG in presurgically implanted patients with epilepsy (Leuthardt et al., 2004, Hinterberger et al., 2008) showed high classification rates of 70–90% accuracy in selecting letters from different speller systems using brain oscillations derived from motor-related areas with frequencies up to the high gamma range without extensive training times. Patients used different types of imagery to select or ignore a particular letter or object from a computer menu. The first implantation of 100 microelectrodes in the motor cortex of a high spinal cord patient by Hochberg, Mukand, Polykoff, Friehs, and Donoghue (2005) seems to allow improved BCI performance. In our laboratory, two patients in CLIS suffering from ALS were implanted with ECoG electrodes after failure to communicate with EEG and pH recordings (Ramos Murguialday et al., 2011; Wilhelm et al., 2006). Despite an already well-trained

P3-based-BCI, a paradigm based on detection of ERPs requiring directed attention in a specific sensory modality (e.g. vision, hearing, touch) that was established during the LIS in one patient, neither of these two patients achieved reliable brain communication rates with ECoG-BCIs. Furthermore, improving the quality and degrees of freedom in the brain signals (e.g., using single cell firing or LFP) was not superior to noninvasive recordings in these CLIS patients (Birbaumer, 2006, Birbaumer et al., 2008). This essentially negative result of invasive brain recording suggests a more fundamental theoretical problem of learning and attention in brain communication with BCI in CLIS. However, the database of invasive BCIs for communication purposes in paralyzed patients at present is too small to judge their efficacy, and the willingness of patients and their families to agree to implantation is weak as long as the noninvasive BCIs are available and functioning.

Noninvasive EEG-based BCI for communication

Three different types of EEG-based BCI are currently in use: namely, slow cortical potential (SCP)-BCI; SMR-BCI; and P3-BCI.

The SCP-BCI

Slow cortical potentials with a negative or positive polarity are recorded as a result of sustained intracortical or thalamocortical input to cortical layers I and II and if negative, indicate simultaneous depolarization of large pools of apical dendrites of pyramidal neurons. The depolarization of cortical cell assemblies reduces their excitation threshold, and firing of neurons in regions responsible for motor or cognitive tasks is facilitated (Birbaumer et al., 1990). These potential shifts occur over 0.5–10.0 seconds. Negative SCPs are typically associated with movement and other functions involving cortical activation, while positive SCPs are usually associated with reduced cortical activation (Rockstroh et al., 1989; Birbaumer, 1999). In studies over more than 30 years, Birbaumer and his colleagues have shown that people can learn to control SCPs and thereby control movement of an object on a computer screen (Elbert et al., 1980, Birbaumer et al., 1999, 2000). This demonstration is the basis for a BCI referred to as a "thought translation device" (TTD). The principal emphasis has been on developing clinical application of this BCI system. It has been tested extensively in people with late-stage ALS and has proved able to supply basic communication capability (Kübler, 2000). For SCP recording, the EEG has to be measured with long time constants of several seconds, and usually feedback from the central Cz electrode is provided. SCPs are extracted by appropriate filtering, corrected for EOG activity, and fed back to the user via visual feedback from a computer screen that shows one choice at the top and one at the bottom. Selection takes four seconds. During a two-second baseline period, the system measures the user's initial voltage level. In the next two seconds, the user selects the top or bottom choice by decreasing or increasing the voltage level by a criterion amount.

The voltage is displayed as vertical movement of a cursor and final selection is indicated in a variety of ways, as shown in Figure 6.2. The BCI can also operate in a mode that gives auditory or tactile feedback (Birbaumer et al., 2000). Over a period of several years in Birbaumer's lab in Tübingen, 25 patients were confronted with SCP-BCI and were trained successfully, from two up to several hundred sessions over weeks, months, or years (as summarized in Table 6.1), to communicate. (Refer to Figure 6.2 in Colour Plate Section)

The SMR-BCI

SMR refers to localized sinusoidal frequencies in the alpha and lower beta range of EEG activity, which can be recorded over somatosensory and motor cortical areas (Niedermeyer, 2005). SMR decreases or desynchronizes with movement, preparation for movement, or movement imagery, and it increases or synchronizes in the post-movement period or during motor quiescence (Pfurtscheller & Aranibar, 1979). Wolpaw and colleagues at the Wadsworth Laboratories in Albany, New York, did an extensive series of experiments, mainly with healthy persons, using SMR rather than SCP as the target brain response (Wolpaw et al., 2002). In a group of patients, two with high spinal cord lesions, Wolpaw and McFarland (2004) demonstrated that multidimensional control of a cursor movement on a computer screen can be learned in just a few sessions of training. The subjects were able to move a cursor within 10 seconds into one of eight goals appearing randomly at one of the four corners of the screen. The flexibility, speed, and learning performance are generally equal to that seen when invasive multielectrode BCI systems are tested in animals. The Wolpaw and McFarland (2004) preparation consisted of a simple electrode montage covering the hand and foot area with a linear online filtering and detection algorithm used for data reduction and quantification. To learn to modulate the power of SMR, patients can receive feedback (e.g., cursor movement on a computer screen in one or two dimensions) (Wolpaw & McFarland, 2004). During each trial of one-dimensional control, patients are presented with one or more targets as shown in Figure 6.2. The patient's task is to move the cursor on the target. For example, low SMR amplitude during motor imagery moves the cursor to the bottom bar, high SMR amplitude moves the cursor toward the top bar (Kübler, Winter, Ludolph et al., 2005). In Birbaumer's lab in Tubingen, patients were trained successfully for communication with SMR–BCI and participated in from nine up to 20 sessions as summarized in Table 6.1.

The P3-BCI

The P3 is a positive deflection of varying amplitude in the EEG. It is typically seen when participants are required to attend to a random sequence of rare (target) and of frequent standard stimuli, an experimental design referred to as "oddball paradigm." In the classic P3-BCI, first introduced by Farwell and Donchin, participants are presented with a 6 × 6 matrix in which each of the 36 cells contains a letter or a symbol (Farwell and Donchin, 1988).

Table 6.1 List of all patients who have been confronted with a BCI since 1995 in the laboratory at the University of Tübingen

Patient	Diagnosis	Age[a]	Sex	Duration of participation/ year of study entry	Level of impairment	Type of BCI and average CRR[b]			Level of success[c]	CRR published in
						SCP	SMR	P300		
HPS	ALS spinal	41	m	Present/1996	4	87		73	4 (SCP), 3 (P300)[f]	Kübler et al. (1999)
JB	ALS bulbar	49	m	2 years/1997	4	86			4 (SCP)	Birbaumer et al. (1999)
MP	ALS spinal	37	m	2 years/1997	3	66			3 (SCP)	Kübler et al. (1999)
MW	Brain stem stroke	26	f	Months/1995	4	X[d]			2 (SCP)	Kübler et al. (1998)
HE	ALS spinal	42	m	Present/1998	3	94			4 (SCP)	Neumann and Birbaumer (2003)
EK	ALS spinal	66	m	Months/1998	2	57			2 (SCP)	Neumann and Birbaumer (2003)
MZ	ALS spinal	31	m	Months/2000	4	70			3 (SCP)	Kübler et al. (2001)
LB	ALS	63	m	Months/1999	5	48			1 (SCP)	Neumann and Birbaumer (2003)
NB	ALS	40	m	Months/2000	5	59			2 (SCP)	Neumann and Birbaumer (2003)
KI	Cerebral paresis	33	m	Months/1998	3	50			1 (SCP)	Kübler (2000)
TK	Muscular dystrophy	33	m	Months/1998/2006	4	43		59	1 (SCP), 2 (P300)[f]	Kübler (2000)
RCS	ALS spinal	56	m	1 year/2003	4		77	69	3 (SMR), 2 (P300)	Kübler et al. (2005) and Nijboer at el. (2008)
HAC	ALS bulbar	67	m	2 years/2003	2		78	86	3 (SMR), 4 (P300)	Kübler et al. (2005) and Nijboer et al. (2008)

(Continued)

Table 6.1 Continued

Patient	Diagnosis	Age[a]	Sex	Duration of participation/ year of study entry	Level of impairment	Type of BCI and average CRR[b] SCP	SMR	P300	Level of success[c]	CRR published in
UBA	ALS spinal	47	f	Present/2004	3		81	82	3 (SMR), 4 (P300)	Kübler et al. (2005) and Nijboer et al. (2008)
HM	ALS spinal	53	m	3 years/2002	2	67	76	32	2 (SCP), 3 (SMR), 2(P300)	Kübler et al. (2004), Kübler et al. (2005) and Nijboer et al. (2008)
JAK	ALS spinal	39	m	2 years/2005	3			50	2 (P300)	Nijboer et al. (2008)
LEK	ALS spinal	49	f	Present/2004	3			80	3(P300)	Nijboer et al. (2008)
IR	ALS spinal	42	f	Present/2003	5	54	43		1 (SCP), 1 (SMR)	Kübler et al. (2004)
SM	ALS spinal	35	m	Months/2002	2	84			3 (SCP)	Kübler et al. (2004)
KW	ALS spinal	47	f	Months/2002	2	78			3 (SCP)	Kübler et al. (2004)
GW	ALS bulbar	59	f	Months/2002	2	70			3 (SCP)	Kübler et al. (2004)
GB	ALS spinal	62	f	Months/2002	2	79			3 (SCP)	Kübler et al. (2004)
KR	ALS spinal	35	f	Present/2002	3	62		87	2 (SCP), 4 (P300)	Kübler et al. (2004) and Nijboer et al. (2008)
HJZ	ALS	60	m	Months/2002	3	74			3 (SCP)	Kübler et al. (2004)
RB	ALS spinal	64	f	Months/2002	1	68			2 (SCP)	Kübler et al. (2004)
JF	ALS spinal	50	m	Months/2002	1	61			2 (SCP)	Kübler et al. (2004)
GR	ALS spinal	37	m	Present/2005	4	74			3 (P300)[ff]	Kübler et al. (2004)
PR	Heart attack	55	m	Years[i]/2002	5	50	X[e]	X[g]	1 (SCP)[f], 1 (SMR), 1 (P300)[f]	Hill et al. (2006)
AG	Chronic GBS[j]	42	f	Years[i]/2000	5	50	X[e]	X[g]	1 (SCP)[f], 1 (SMR), 1 (P300)f	Hill et al. (2006)
WER	ALS spinal	63	m	Days/2005	5		X[e]	X[g]	1 (SMR), 1 (P300)[f]	Hill et al. (2006)
G	Stroke	61	m	One session/2005	4		X[e]		1 (SMR)	Hill et al. (2006)

Patient	Diagnosis	Age	Sex	Duration of participation/ year of study entry	Level of impairment	Type of BCI (CS NIRS)	Level of success	CRR published in
WEW	ALS spinal	46	m	Months/2004	4	X[g]	1 (P300)	Nijboer et al. (2008)
EM	ALS spinal	58	m	Weeks/2002	5	62	2 (SCP)	Hinterberger et al. (2005)
VWI	ALS spinal	57	f	3 Sessions/2007	4	63	2 (P300)[f]	
UB	ALS spinal		m	Months/1997	2	X[h]		
Pat. 1	ALS spinal and sporadic	66	f	37 days/2012 (CS), 14 days/2013 (NIRS)	CLIS	CS NIRS	50% (CS), 71.67% (NIRS)	De Massari et al. (2013) and Gallegos-Ayala et al. (2014)
Pat. 2	ALS bulbar	72	m	2 Weeks/2012		CS	48%	De Massari et al. (2013)
Pat. 3	ALS spinal	40	m	2 Weeks/2012		CS	58%	De Massari et al. (2013)

a   Age at study entry.

b   Average over three representative sessions or as reported in publication. If more than one CRR was available (in different publications), the highest published CRR was chosen.

c   The highest level of success was chosen for analysis regardless of type of BCI.

d   *Above chance level* performance, but CRR not reported in publication.

e   Chance level performance in first training session and no further SMR–BCI training was conducted; CRR not reported in publication.

f   Unpublished.

g   No P300 detectable, and thus no training with the P300–BCI was conducted.

h   Data lost due to trainer error.

i   With interruptions.

j   Guillain–Barré Syndrome.

This design becomes an oddball paradigm by first intensifying each row and column for 100 ms in random order and then by instructing participants to attend to only one (the desired) of the 36 cells. Thus, in one trial of 12 flashes (6 rows and 6 columns), the target cell will flash only twice, constituting a rare event compared to the 10 flashes of all other rows and columns, and will therefore elicit a P300 (Sellers and Donchin, 2006) (Figure 6.2). In the study by Sellers and Donchin, 11 ALS patients were trained with a P3-BCI and participated in from three up to 60 sessions. Eight patients were trained with two types and three patients with all three types of BCI (Table 6.1). BCI training was conducted between one and three times a week.

Based on the detailed comparison of three different signatures of EEG-based BCIs as reported in Birbaumer (2006), it was concluded that in ALS patients with functioning vision and eye control, SMR-BCI and P3-BCI show the most promising results. SCP-BCIs need more extensive training than other BCIs but may have the best stability and are more independent of the sensory, motor, and cognitive functioning necessary for their application in LIS and CLIS patients. The patients described earlier (Birbaumer, 1999) had high success rates with SCP-BCI training, but only after many sessions. It has been postulated that some cognitive impairment and changes in EEG signatures in late-stage ALS may contribute to the lack of success using EEG-BCI technology as the technology was introduced after the participants had become CLIS (Munte et al., 1998). Kübler and Birbaumer (2008) have shown that patients in CLIS do not reach sufficient BCI control for communication with EEG parameters. Kübler and Birbaumer (2008) speculated that extinction of goal-directed thinking may prohibit operant learning of brain communication. The most successful application for communication has occurred in people at the early stages of the disease (Birbaumer et. al, 1999; Birbaumer, 2006; Kübler et al., 2001). Hence, there is a need to find an alternative learning paradigm and probably another neuroimaging technique to design a more effective BCI to help ALS patient in CLIS with communication.

Complete paralysis and CLIS requires alternative BCI-paradigms

CLIS caused by destruction or degeneration of the motor system in ALS, or due to brain stem stroke or other types of brain damage and diseases, is usually accompanied by changes in circadian rhythm, sleep pattern, and arousal with alterations of attentional performance (Ramos Murguialday et al., 2011). These changes may be at least partially responsible for BCI communication failures. While in LIS with intact eye control and other states of incomplete paralysis circadian rhythm is irregular, sleep polysomnographic recordings over several nights in one CLIS patient with implanted ECoG-electrodes showed chaotic sleep patterns with unpredictable slow wave sleep episodes during the day. BCI sessions usually are scheduled during daytime hours, without polysomnographic recordings and without online detection of sleep. Fading vigilance during learning of BCI-based communication methods may be an inevitable consequence, because sleep cannot be detected behaviorally by any means in a motionless, artificially-respirated CLIS patient whose eyes are closed, except through analysis of EEG signals (Birbaumer et al., 2014).

The lack of reliable brain communication, even with invasive recordings, in CLIS patients (Ramos Murguialday et al., 2011) is mirrored by the complete failure of noninvasive EEG-BCIs to reinstate communication in complete paralysis. A meta-analysis of all reported ALS patients by Kübler and Birbaumer (2008) and a longitudinal study by Silvoni et al. (2013) indicate that noninvasive BCIs based on imagery or instrumental-operant learning (Birbaumer et al., 1999) did not achieve sufficient communication rates and performance of BCI, failing to meet a 70%-correct threshold for sufficient online classification of "yes" or "no" responses (select–reject) and, thus, are also difficult to apply for differential diagnosis between CLIS and VS/UWS. Birbaumer et al. (2012) hypothesized that "loss of the contingency between a voluntary response and its feedback" or loss of subsequent reward in individuals who are completely paralyzed would prevent learning, even if auditory afferent input and cognitive processing (attention, memory, imagery) remained intact. If the voluntary response is cognitive, such as in covert goal-orientated imagery in the LIS, the feedback or reward does not follow a reliable environmental or internal change and the response consequently extinguishes. Psychophysical studies (Haggard et al., 2002) demonstrate that, if the behavioral response is elicited independently of a conscious decision and intention, the conscious awareness of the contingency and the conscious experience of the decision (the "will") vanish. In CLIS, contingencies between goal-directed thinking and intentions are lost because there is no environmental response to the particular intention. This process was termed as the "extinction of goal directed thinking" or "extinction of thought." A single case of a CLIS patient able to communicate with a BCI based on instrumental (voluntary) learning and training after entering that state without a history of BCI control would disprove this speculation. In the BCI literature, or in the literature of LIS and in extensive studies of operant physiological regulation in the curarized rat (Dworkin and Miller, 1986), no such case has yet been reported.

A possible way to address the "extinction of thought" problem and prevent extinction may be to create artificial contingencies. For example, it would be possible to utilize transcranial magnetic stimulation pulses or peripheral nerve stimulation applied to a specific body part or to different frontal or motor brain areas contingent on the elicited brain response or contingent on peripheral nerve responses of the BCI. Extensive successful BCI training should also prevent cessation of brain communication if the BCI response can be maintained in the CLIS. However, none of our ALS patients proficient in BCI control ever passed from LIS to CLIS, which may suggest that the S-E-R (stimulus [S], response [R], and effect [E]) contingency and communication provided by the BCI may exert a neuroprotective effect. This speculation, however, is difficult to substantiate. We believe that the absence of extensive contingent stimulation and reward during waking hours may lead to the loss of associative connections between intention to communicate and response or consequence. Transmission of external currents and magnetic fields into the brain to induce or accelerate learning of BCI control may also represent an interesting future extension of existing BCI systems (see Karim, Kammer, Cohen, & Birbaumer, 2004, for a first attempt).

Another possibility to address these problems may include metabolic BCIs using fMRI or NIRS (see Sitaram et al., 2007a, b). Metabolic changes and vascular variations are sensed by arterial receptors and may be utilized to control contingent reafferent perceptual responses (Adam, 1998). However, evidence so far indicates that even metabolic brain activity needs a history of learned contingencies in order to be evoked voluntarily and to become useful for communication in the CLIS. It is still unclear whether successful BCI training can be transferred from the partially LIS to the CLIS. The only case described in the literature by our lab (Ramos Murguialday et al., 2011) failed to achieve reliable BCI communication despite implantation of ECoG electrodes epidurally.

Classical "Reflexive" conditioning for BCI communication

After failure to replicate operant physiological regulation in the curarized paralyzed rat, Dworkin (1993) proved successful classical conditioning of various physiological responses (i.e., firing rate of facial nerves), of completely paralyzed rats. Stimulus–Stimulus (S–S) conditioning does not rely on goal-directed voluntary-operant motor preparation and response execution. Based on these animal experiments (Birbaumer et al., 2008; Birbaumer and Cohen, 2007), classical semantic conditioning was attempted in several ALS patients in LIS and one CLIS patient. Classical semantic conditioning in humans was extensively demonstrated by Pavlov's students and summarized by Razran (1961). Commonly, during classical conditioning a neutral conditioned stimulus (CS) is repeatedly paired with a biologically relevant (e.g., aversive) unconditioned stimulus (US). Once a CS–US association has been formed, the CS produces a conditioned reaction (CR) in anticipation of the US. No voluntary-operant response effort is required in classical "reflex" conditioning, and only minimal semantic priming is necessary in classical conditioning. Therefore, this approach might reopen a remaining communication pathway in patients with more or less severe cognitive disorders as reported previously (Ludolphet et al., 1992; Volpato et al., 2010). Semantic classical conditioning refers to conditioning of a physiological or behavioral response to a meaningful word or sentence irrespective of the particular constituent letters or sounds of the words (Razran, 1961). Originated in Russian research of the 1950s and 1960s, semantic conditioning is based on generalization of CRs along a semantic dimension (word-to-word transfer). It has been shown that CRs (e.g., saliva secretion, galvanic skin response, heart rate) to specific words or sentences can be transferred to other words or sentences with similar meaning (Razran, 1939, 1949a, 1949b; Lacey and Smith, 1954). Additionally, there are evidences for cortical correlates of semantic classical conditioning showing that words associated with aversive stimuli (through frequent pairing) evoke stronger cortical responses compared with words not associated with pain or discomfort (Montoya et al., 1996). Thus, during the classical semantic conditioning, words or sentences belonging to different semantic categories were presented as conditioned stimuli (CS). One specific semantic category (i.e., the thought "no") was followed by an unconditioned stimulus (US), usually a non-painful electric shock. Differential conditioning, generalization to semantically related CSs, and extinction of diverse physiological responses were reported (Razran, 1961). Obviously, classical semantic conditioning of autonomic responses or brain responses does not depend on goal-directed motor systems and involves only minimal attentional resources and effort. Thus, classical semantic conditioning may circumvent extinction of volition, goal-directed thinking, effortful selective attention, and cognitive control, imagery, and working memory functions during operant learning and, thus, represent a principle to maintain communication in complete paralysis. These predictions were evaluated in a series of experiments involving healthy participants and ALS patients at various stages of their disease, all of them in LIS or CLIS (Furdea et al., 2012; Ruf et al., 2013; De Massari et al., 2013). Patients suffering from ALS in the advanced stage were artificially fed and artificially respirated. The complete paralysis was verified through repetitive recordings of eye movements and electromyographic recordings from various muscles over a period of several weeks (Ramos Murguialday et al., 2011). No control of external sphincter or eye was present and all patients were incontinent. Because paralysis of eye movements is frequently accompanied by loss of clear vision due to drying of the cornea and eyeball, only the auditory and tactile modality remains for interactive purposes, although extended bed rest and skin deformations may also compromise tactile and somatosensory input channels as documented previously (Ramos Murguialday et al., 2011). Lack of any type of communication with the patients was verified by relatives and nursing personnel and documented in repeated video recordings. Online classification of different components of EEG oscillations and ERP signals associated with "yes" or "no" responses was performed (see Figure 6.3). De Massari et al. (2013), for example, reported 37 sessions of classical semantic conditioning in one CLIS patient (and eight sessions in two LIS patients) using wavelet classification and nonlinear support vector machines (SVM) of fronto-central SCP to "yes" and "no" questions, resulting in correct classification above 70% in some sessions. After training of the classifier based on several hundred questions with well-known answers (e.g., "Rome is the capital of Germany"), personal and open questions (e.g., "you want to be turned to . . .") were presented. While useful communication needs at least 70% correct classification of brain signals over an extended period of sessions (Birbaumer, Kübler, Ghanayim et al., 2000), in the reported CLIS patient only seven out of 37 sessions resulted in sufficient classification (De Massari et al., 2013). A particular challenge is the validation of answers to open questions, as validation often depends on family members and long-term nursing personnel introducing biases towards their own expectations. Frequent repetition of semantically differently phrased questions over days and weeks (i.e., "you are not in constant pain," instead of "you are in constant pain") might help to control for this problem. Thus, although the classical conditioning paradigm showed potential, the EEG could not be used reliably for successful communication.

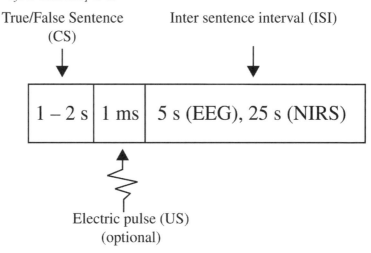

Figure 6.3 Principle of the semantic classical conditioning BCI. (Figure from Birbaumer et al., 2013)

Metabolic BCI

fMRI-based BCI for ALS patients

Functional magnetic resonance imaging measures increases and decreases of paramagnetic load of blood flow to activated pools of neurons, particularly to apical dendrites (Logothetis et al., 2001). Paramagnetic charge is determined by blood oxygenation level-dependent (BOLD) flow, which reflects local metabolic deficiencies of the vascular bed supplying the neurons. Logothetis et al., 2001, have shown that the correlation of local blood flow change and the BOLD signal is particularly high for the neuronal inflow to the apical dendrites reflecting primarily intracortical activity. The fMRI-based BCI is difficult to apply in severely motor-disabled patients because it is expensive, bulky, and impossible to move to patients' homes. Moreover, the patient enclosed in the scanner does not experience a satisfying environment for communication. Still, instrumental learning of BOLD control turned out to be successful in some neuropsychiatric disorders such as unipolar depression (Linden et al., 2012; Birbaumer, Ruiz & Sitaram, 2013), psychopathology (Sitaram et al., 2007a; Birbaumer et al., 2005), paranoid schizophrenia (Ruiz et al., 2013), and nicotine dependency (Li et al., 2013).

NIRS-based BCI for ALS patients

NIRS is an emerging neuroimaging modality that employs near-infrared light to noninvasively or invasively investigate cerebral oxygenation changes in healthy and neurologically impaired adults and children (Stragmann et al., 2002). It has reasonable spatial and good temporal resolution and is relatively robust to motion artifact, thereby enabling it to be suitable for investigating everyday tasks. Thus, in contrast to fMRI, a NIRS-based BCI can easily be applied at the bedside of highly impaired patients who are difficult to move and in desperate need for communication.

Sitaram et al. (2007b) published the first controlled evaluation of a NIRS-BCI. Using motor imagery with a 20-channel NIRS system over sensorimotor cortex, they reported 89% correct classification of right- and left-hand motor imagery without any training and the use of a hidden Markov model as a classifier. Recently, we demonstrated stable brain communication with NIRS using the classical conditioning procedure in a CLIS patient (Gallegos-Ayala et al., 2014) who was previously trained with an EEG-BCI (De Massari et al., 2013). While EEG-BCI application resulted in significant (above 70%) classification of "yes" and "no" responses in only seven of 37 sessions and no discriminatory response in brain oscillations at frequencies between 3 Hz and 30 Hz, NIRS-BCI communication resulted in an overall stability of 72% – 100% correct answers across 14 consecutive sessions (Figure 6.4). Blood oxygenation from frontal to central sensors increased during 25 seconds of "yes"-thinking and decreased during "no"-thinking. This clinical experiment is the first demonstration of stable BCI-based communication using semantic classical conditioning in a CLIS patient. This result holds promise and raises hope for communication in CLIS.

Hence, to further validate these preliminary findings of our lab and to refine the technology of NIRS-based BCI for communication in CLIS patients, extensive studies are presently being carried out on several CLIS patients using combined NIRS-EEG-based BCIs. (Refer to Figure 6.4 in Colour Plate Section)

Ethical considerations of BCI in complete paralysis

Current legal systems in most industrialized countries provide the possibility to declare a "patient will" or "advanced directive" in case of medical emergencies. The patients' will declarations can include the patient's wish that "artificial" life-preserving medical interventions, such as artificial respiration and feeding and similar intensive care measures, would be prohibitive and should be avoided. In most cases, however, these patients' wills are signed long before such a medical emergency occurs. The underlying assumption of the signing persons (and these documents) is very often that the circumstances requiring life-preserving measures are associated with a poor quality of life. In contrast to this widespread assumption, well-controlled studies in patients with LIS, ALS, chronic stroke, and other chronic and untreatable neurological diseases show average and sometimes above average quality of life (Lulé et al., 2009; Kübler, Nijboer, Mellinger et al., 2005, 2006, 2008), despite paralysis and artificial respiration and feeding. Still, about 95% of all ALS patients in most industrialized countries "choose" to die before tracheostromy and artificial respiration. Widespread hidden euthanasia is the rule and not the exception for these patients. In places with "liberalization" of assisted suicide and euthanasia, such as The Netherlands, Belgium, and

Oregon, more patients choose death before emergency measures are taken than in countries with less "liberal" euthanasia laws such as Germany and Israel. This underscores the fact that "patients' will"-declarations are probably invalid at the decisive time points. They may serve as an excuse for the medical professions, insurance systems, or family members to shorten anticipated long periods of care for these patients and avoid the financial and social burdens. Patients themselves may follow the social pressure and accept the poor quality-of-life prognosis and ask for hastened death. If quality of life is measured objectively in the absence of doctors and family members, a significant difference between quality-of-life estimation by the patient and others may emerge. Some paralyzed and respirated ALS patients judge their quality of life as satisfactory and good, while others may attribute very poor quality of life and depression to the motionless patient (Kübler, Nijboer, Mellinger et al., 2005; Lulé et al., 2012; Matuz et al., 2010; Pantke and Birbaumer, 2012). The CLIS patient that Gallegos-Ayala et al. (2014) describe was completely paralyzed for 20 months without any ability to communicate, artificially respirated, and fed over three years. This patient articulated, with the help of the BCI-system, good mood and good quality of life. While single case reports do not provide scientific proof, a more extreme case than this is difficult to imagine in modern medicine. This case strengthens the need to conduct more controlled studies with patients in these severe and/or less severe conditions. In a broader study from Bruno et al. (2011), 168 patients were invited to participate in a survey about their quality of life. Ninety-one patients (54%) responded, and 26 were excluded because of missing data. Out of the 65 remaining patients, 47 declared being happy and 18 were unhappy. A current wish for euthanasia was expressed by four of the 59 subjects who answered the question (7%). Interestingly, variables associated with unhappiness included dissatisfaction with mobility in the community, with recreational activities, and with the capacity to deal with life events. In our view, and given these findings, shortening-of-life requests by LIS patients are valid and should be heard. However, it is important to give them a chance to achieve a steady state of subjective life-being before any decisions are made. This could partly be achieved by developing efficient BCI to communicate with and offer more independence to this population. Therefore, it is worthwhile to further investigate semantic classical conditioning for BCI communication in CLIS. While there is no evidence that invasive BCIs had any advantage over noninvasive systems when using the commonly-used BCI paradigms (Ramos Murguialday et al., 2011), it is conceivable that novel paradigms might change this assessment. However, various ethical considerations must be taken into account when implanting invasive BCIs in patients who are unable to give informed consent. Most legal systems (e.g., in Germany) require that the relatives or legal guardians allow implantation but do not require consent by an ethics committee. This regulation acts on the assumption that relatives or legal guardians are able to reconstruct the patient's will based on their acquaintance with the person. It also assumes that the relatives or legal guardians decide in the interest of the patient. The availability of BCI technology yielding the described study results may force us to deny hastened death requests formulated in patient wills or advance directives signed long before the present state of a disease. We do not, however, generally deny the right of a person in a particular state of an intractable and often painful disease such as terminal cancer to ask for and receive death in dignity and without pain. The unresolved ethical problems associated with the advancements in neurotechnology and BCI research urge a broad and open-minded societal discourse (Vlek et al., 2012; Clausen 2008, 2009; for more discussion about this topic in disorders of consciousness, see Chapter 7).

Acknowledgments

We acknowledge the participation of all our patients, particularly of Joachim Faehnrich, Sonja Hunger, and the family of Blauwitz, the family of Gröschel, and the family of Kerstin Wirth. Because of them we have been able to shed light on the use of BCI in CLIS-ALS patients. We also thank all of the researchers who were part of the team at different stages of the research as well as our funding sources: Deutsche Forschungsgemeinschaft (DFG, Kosellek), Stiftung Volkswagenwerk (VW), Brain Products, Gilching and German Center of Diabetes Research (DZD) at the University of Tübingen, Eva and Horst Köhler Stiftung, and Baden-Württernberg-Stiftung.

Notes

1 **Ujwal Chaudhary** is a postdoctoral research fellow at the Institute for Medical Psychology and Behavioral Neurobiology, Eberhard-Karls-University of Tübingen, Germany.
2 **Francesco Piccione** is the Director of Medical Neurology at the Istituto di Ricovero e Cura a carattere scientifico (IRCCS), Ospedale San Camillo, Venice, Italy.
3 **Niels Birbaumer** is a professor at the Institute for Medical Psychology and Behavioral Neurobiology, Eberhard-Karls-University of Tübingen, Germany.

References

Abeles, M. (1991). *Corticonics: Neural Circuits of the Cerebral Cortex*. New York: Cambridge University Press.

Adam, G. (1998). *Visceral Perception*. New York: Plenum Press.

Aggarwal, A., & Nicholson, G. (2002). Detection of preclinical motor neuron loss in SOD-1 mutation carriers using motor unit number estimation. *J Neurol Neurosurg Psychiatry*, 73(2), 199–201.

Ball, L., Beukelman, D., & Bardach, L. (2007). AAC intervention for ALS. In: D. Beukelman, K. Garrett, & K. Yorkston, Eds. *Augmentative Communication Strategies for Adults with Acute or Chronic Medical Conditions*. Baltimore: Paul H. Brookes, pp. 287–316.

Bauer, G., Gerstenbrand, F., & Rumpl, E. (1979). Varieties of the locked-in syndrome, *J Neurol*, 221(2), 77–91.

Beleza-Meireles, A., & Al-Chalabi, A. (2009). Genetic studies of amyotrophic lateral sclerosis: controversies and perspectives. *Amyotroph Lateral Scler*, 10(1), 1–14.

Beukelman, D., & Mirenda, P. (2005). *Augmentative and Alternative Communication: Supporting Children Adults with Complex Communication Needs.* Baltimore: Paul H. Brookes.

Birbaumer, N., Elbert, T., Canavan, A. G. M., & Rockstroh, B. (1990). Slow potentials of the cerebral cortex and behavior. *Physiol Rev*, 70(1), 1–41.

Birbaumer, N. (1999). Slow cortical potentials: their origin, meaning, and clinical use. In: G. J. M. van Boxtel & K. B. E. Böcker, Eds. *Brain and Behavior Past, Present, and Future.* Tilburg: Tilburg University Press, pp. 25–39.

Birbaumer, N., Ghanayim, N., Hinterberger, T., Iversen, I., Kotchoubey, B., Kübler, A., Perelmouter, J., Taub, E., & Flor, H. (1999). A spelling device for the paralyzed. *Nature*, 398, 297–298.

Birbaumer, N., Kübler, A., Ghanayim, N., Hinterberger, T., Perelmouter, J., Kaiser, J., Iversen, I., Kotchoubey, B., Neumann, N., & Flor, H. (2000). The thought translation device (TTD) for completely paralyzed patients. *IEEE Trans Rehabil Eng*, 11(2), 120–123.

Birbaumer, N., Veit, R., Lotze, M., Erb, M., Hermann, C., Grodd, W., & Flor, H. (2005). Deficient fear conditioning in psychopathy: a functional magnetic resonance imaging study. *Arch Gen Psychiatry*, 62(7), 799–805.

Birbaumer, N. (2006). Brain-computer-interface research: coming of age. *Clinical Neurophysiology*, 117(3), 479–483.

Birbaumer, N., & Cohen, L. G. (2007). Brain-computer interfaces: communication and restoration of movement in paralysis. *J Physiol*, 579(3), 621–636.

Birbaumer, N., Murguialday, A. R., & Cohen, L. (2008). Brain computer interface in paralysis. *Curr Opin Neurol*, 21(6), 634–638.

Birbaumer, N., Piccione, F., Silvoni, S., & Wildgruber, M. (2012). Ideomotor silence: the case of complete paralysis and brain-computer interfaces (BCI). *Psychol Res*, 76(2), 183–191.

Birbaumer, N., Gallegos-Ayala, G., Wildgruber, M., Silvoni, S., & Soekadar, S. R. (2014). Direct brain control and communication in paralysis. *Brain Topogr*, 27(1), 4–11.

Birbaumer, N., Ruiz, S., & Sitaram, R. (2013). Learned regulation of brain metabolism. *Trends in Cognitive Sciences*, 17(6), 295–302.

Brunner, C., Graimann, B., Huggins, J. E., Levine, S. P., & Pfurtscheller, G. (2005). Phase relationships between different subdural electrode recordings in man. *Neuroscience Letters*, 375(2), 69–74.

Bruno, M. A., Bernheim, J. L., Ledoux, D., Pellas, F., Demertzi, A., & Laureys, S. (2011). A survey on self-assessed well-being in a cohort of chronic locked-in syndrome patients: happy majority, miserable minority. *BMJ Open*, 1(1), e000039.

Caria, A., Veit, R., Sitaram, R., Lotze, M., Weiskopf, N., Grodd, W., Birbaumer, N. (2007). Regulation of anterior insular cortex activity using real-time fMRI. *NeuroImage*, 35(3), 1238–1246.

Clausen, J. (2008). Moving minds: ethical aspects of neural motor prostheses. *Biotechnol J*, 3(12), 1493–1501.

Clausen, J. (2009). Man, machine and in between. *Nature*, 457, 1080–1081.

de Carvalho, M., & Swash, M. (2006). The onset of amyotrophic lateral sclerosis. *J Neurol Neurosurg Psychiatry*, 77, 388–389.

De Massari, D., Matuz, T., Furdea, A., Ruf, C. A., Halder, S., & Birbaumer, N. (2013). Brain-computer interface and semantic classical conditioning of communication in paralysis. *Biol Psychol*, 92(2), 267–274.

Deng, H. X., Zhai, H., Bigio, E. H., Yan, J., Fecto, F., Ajroud, K., Mishra, M., Ajroud-Driss, S., Heller, S., Sufit, R., Siddique, N., Mugnaini, E., & Siddique, T. (2010). FUS-immunoreactive inclusions are a common feature in sporadic and non-SOD1 familial amyotrophic lateral sclerosis. *Ann Neurol*, 67(6), 739–748.

Donaghy, C., Pinnock, R., Abrahams, S., Cardwell, C., Hardiman, O., Patterson, V., McGivern, R. C., & Gibson, J. M. (2009). Ocular fixation instabilities in motor neurone disease. *J Neurol*, 256(3), 420–426.

Donaghy, C., Pinnock, R., Abrahams, S., Cardwell, C., Hardiman, O., Patterson, V., McGivern, R. C., & Gibson, J. M. (2010). Slow saccades in bulbar-onset motor neurone disease. *J Neurol*, 257(7), 1134–1140.

Dworkin, B. R., & Miller, N. E. (1986). Failure to replicate visceral learning in the acute curarized rat preparation. *Behav Neurosci*, 100(3), 299–314.

Dworkin, B. R. (1993). *Learning and physiological regulation.* Chicago: University of Chicago Press.

Eisen, A., Kim, S. & Pant, B. (1992). Amyotrophic lateral sclerosis (ALS): a phylogenetic disease of the corticomotoneuron? *Muscle Nerve*, 15(2), 219–224.

Elbert, T., Rockstroh, B., Lutzenberger, W., & Birbaumer, N. (1980). Biofeedback of slow cortical potentials. *Electroenceph clin Neurophysiol*, 48(3), 293–301.

Farwell, L. A., & Donchin, E. (1988). Talking off the top of your head: toward a mental prosthesis utilizing event-related brain potentials. *Electroencephalogr Clin Neurophysiol*, 70(6), 512–23.

Felton, E. A., Wilson, J. A., Williams, J. C., & Garell, P. C. (2007). Electrocorticographically controlled brain-computer interfaces using motor and sensory imagery in patients with temporary subdural electrode implants. *Journal of Neurosurgery*, 106(3), 495–500.

Furdea, A., Ruf, C., Halder, S., De Massari, D., Bogdan, M., Rosenstiel, W., Matuz, T., & Birbaumer, N. (2012). A new (semantic) reflexive brain computer interface: in search for a suitable classifier. *J Neurosci Methods*, 203(1), 233–240.

Gallegos-Ayala, G., Furdea, A., Takano, K., Ruf, C. A., Flor, H., & Birbaumer, N. (2014). Brain communication in a completely locked-in patient using bedside near-infrared spectroscopy. *Neurology*, 82(21), 1930–1932.

Graimann, B., Huggins, J. E., Levine, S. P., & Pfurtscheller, G. (2004). Toward a direct brain interface based on human subdural recordings and wavelet-packet analysis. *IEEE Transactions on Biomedical Engineering*, 51(6), 954–962.

Haggard, P., Clark, S., & Kalogeras, J. (2002). Voluntary action and conscious awareness. *Nat Neurosci*, 5, 382–385.

Hill, N. J., Lal, T. N., Schroder, M., Hinterberger, T., Wilhelm, B., Nijboer, F., Mochty, U., Widman, G., Elger, C. E., Scholkopf, B., Kübler, A., & Birbaumer, N. (2006). Classifying EEG and ECoG signals without subject training for fast BCI implementation: comparison of nonparalyzed and completely paralyzed subjects. *IEEE Trans Neural Syst Rehabil Eng*, 14(2), 183–186.

Hinterberger, T., Birbaumer, N., & Flor, H. (2005). Assessment of cognitive function and communication ability in a completely locked-in patient. *Neurology*, 64(7), 1307–1308.

Hinterberger, T., Widmann, G., Lal, T. N., Hill, J., Tangermann, M., Rosenstiel, W., Schölkopf, B., Elger, C., & Birbaumer, N. (2008). Voluntary brain regulation and communication with electrocorticogram signals. *Epilepsy & Behavior*, 13(2), 300–306.

Hochberg, L.R., Mukand, J.A., Polykoff, G.I., Friehs, G.M., & Donoghue, J.P. (2005). Braingate neuromotor prosthesis: nature and use of neural control signals. *Society for Neuroscience*, Program No. 520.17.

Jackson, A., Mavoori, J., & Fetz, E. (2006). Long-term motor cortex plasticity induced by an electronic neural implant. *Nature*, 444, 56–60.

Karim, A.A., Kammer, T., Cohen, L., & Birbaumer, N. (2004). Effects of TMS and tDCS on the physiological regulation of cortical excitability in a brain-computer interface. *Biomedizinische Technik*, 49, 55–57.

Kennedy, P.R., Kirby, M.T., Moore, M.M., King, B., & Mallory, A. (2004). Computer control using human intracortical local field potentials. *IEEE Transactions on Neural Systems and Rehabilitation Engineering*, 12(3), 339–344.

Kiernan, M.C., Vucic, S., Cheah, B.C., Turner, M.R., Eisen, A., Hardiman, O., Burrell, J.R., Zoing, M.C. (2011). Amyotrophic lateral sclerosis. *Lancet* 377(9769), 942–955.

Kübler, A. (2000). *Brain-Computer Communication – Development of a Brain-Computer Interface for Locked-in Patients on the Basis of the Psychophysiological Self-Regulation Training of Slow Cortical Potentials (SCP)*. Tübingen: Schwäbische Verlagsgesellschaft.

Kübler, A., Kotchoubey, B., Salzmann, H.P., Ghanayim, N., Perelmouter, J., Homberg, V., & Birbaumer, N. (1998). Self-regulation of slow cortical potentials in completely paralyzed human patients. *Neurosci Lett*, 252(3), 171–174.

Kübler, A., Kotchoubey, B., Hinterberger, T., Ghanayim, N., Perelmouter, J., Schauer, M., Fritsch, C., Taub, E., & Birbaumer, N. (1999). The thought translation device: a neurophysiological approach to communication in total motor paralysis. *Exp Brain Res*, 124, 223–232.

Kübler, A., Neumann, N., Kaiser, J., Kotchoubey, B., Hinterberger, T., & Birbaumer, N. (2001). Brain-computer communication: self-regulation of slow cortical potentials for verbal communication. *Arch Phys Med Rehabil*, 82(11), 1533–1539.

Kübler, A., Neumann, N., Wilhelm, B., Hinterberger, T., & Birbaumer, N. (2004). Predictability of brain–computer communication. *J Psychophysiol*, 18(2/3), 121–129.

Kübler, A., Nijboer, F., Mellinger, J., Vaughan, T.M., Pawelzik, H., Schalk, G., McFarland D.J., Birbaumer, N., & Wolpaw, J.R. (2005). Patients with ALS can use sensorimotor rhythms to operate a brain-computer interface. *Neurology*, 64(10), 1775–1777.

Kübler, A., Winter, S., Ludolph, A.C., Hautzinger, M., & Birbaumer, N. (2005). Severity of depressive symptoms and quality of life in patients with amyotrophic lateral sclerosis. *Neurorehabil Neural Repair*, 19(3), 182–193.

Kübler, A., Weber, C., & Birbaumer, N. (2006). Locked-in-freigegeben für den tod? Wenn nur denken und fühlen bleiben – neuroethik des eingeschlossenseins. *Zeitschrift fürmedizinische Ethik*, 52, 57–70.

Kübler, A., & Birbaumer, N. (2008). Brain-computer interfaces and communication in paralysis: extinction of goal directed thinking in completely paralysed patients? *Clinical Neurophysiology*, 119(11), 2658–2666.

Lacey, J., & Smith, R. (1954). Conditioning and generalization of unconscious anxiety. *Science* 120, 1045–1052.

Lebedev, M.A., & Nicolelis, M.A. (2006). Brain machine interfaces: past, present and future. *Trends in Neurosciences*, 29(9), 536–546.

Leuthardt, E.C., Schalk, B., Wolpaw, J.R., Ojemann, J.G., & Moran, D.W. (2004). A brain-computer interface using electrocorticographic signals in humans. *J Neural Eng*, 1(2), 63–71.

Li, X., Hartewell, K.J., Borckardt, J., Prisciandaro, J.J., Saladin, M.E., Morgan, P.S., Johnson, K.A., LeMatty, T., Brady, K.T., & George, M.S. (2013). Volitional reduction of anterior cingulate cortex activity produces decreased cue craving in smoking cessation: a preliminary real-time fMRI study. *Addict Biol*, 18(4), 739–748.

Linden, D. E., Habes, I., Johnston, S. J., Linden, S., Tatineni, R., Subramanian, L., Sorger, B., Healy, D., & Goebel, R. (2012). Real-time self-regulation of emotion networks in patients with depression. *PLoS ONE*, 7(6), e38115.

Logothetis, N., Pauls, J., Augath, M., Trinath, T., & Oeltermann, A. (2001). Neurophysiological investigation of the basis of the fMRI signal. *Nature*, 412, 150–157.

Logroscino, G., Traynor, B. J., Hardiman, O., Chio, A., Mitchell, D., Swinger, R. J., Millul, A., Benn, E., & Beghi, E. (2010). Incidence of amyotrophic lateral sclerosis in Europe. *J Neurol Neurosurg Psychiatry*, 81, 385–390.

Ludolph, A. C., Langen, K., Regard, M., Herzog, H., Kemper, B., Kuwert, T., Böttger, I., & Feinendegen, L. (1992). Frontal lobe function in amyotrophic lateral sclerosis: a neuropsychologic and positron emission tomography study. *Acta Neurologica Scandinavica*, 85(2), 81–89.

Lulé, D., Zickler, C., Bruno, M. A., Demertzi, A., Pellas, F., Laureys, S., & Kübler, A. (2009). Life can be worth living in locked-in syndrome. *Prog Brain Res*, 177, 339–351.

Lulé, D., Pauli, S., Altintas, E., Singer, U., Merk, T., Uttner I., Birbaumer, N., & Ludolph A.C. (2012). Emotional adjustment in amyotrophic lateral sclerosis (ALS). *J Neurol*, 259(2), 334–341.

Matuz, T., Birbaumer, N., Hautzinger, M., & Kübler, A. (2010). Coping with amyotrophic lateral sclerosis: an integrative view. *J Neurol Neurosurg Psychiatry*, 81, 893–898.

Munte, T.F., Troger, M.C., Nusser, I., Wieringa B.M., Johannes, S., Matzke, M., & Dengler, R. (1998). Alteration of early components of the visual evoked potential in amyotrophic lateral sclerosis. *J Neurol*, 245(4), 206–210.

Montoya, P., Larbig, W., Pulvermüller, F., Flor, H., & Birbaumer, N. (1996). Cortical correlates of semantic classical conditioning. *Psychophysiology*, 33(6), 644–649.

Neumann, N., & Birbaumer, N. (2003). Predictors of successful self control during brain–computer communication. *J Neurol Neurosurg Psychiatry*, 74, 1117–1121.

Niedermeyer, E. (2005). The normal EEG of the waking adult. In: E. Niedermeyer & F.H. Lopes da Silva, Eds. *Electroencephalography: Basic Principles, Clinical Applications, and Related Fields*. Philadelphia: Lippincott, pp. 167–192.

Nijboer, F., Furdea, A., Gunst, I., Mellinger, J., McFarland, D. J., Birbaumer. N., & Kübler, A. (2008). An auditory brain-computer-interface (BCI). *J Neurosci Methods*, 167(1), 43–50.

Nijboer, F., Sellers, E. W., Mellinger, J., Jordan, M. A., Matuz, T., Halder, S., Mochty, U., Krusienski, D. J., Vaughan, T. M., Wolpaw, J. R., Birbaumer, N., & Kübler, A. (2008). A P300-based brain-computer interface for people with amyotrophic lateral sclerosis. *Clinical Neurophysiology*, 119(8), 1909–1916.

Norris, F. H. (1992). Amyotrophic lateral sclerosis: the clinical disorder. In: R. A. Smith, Ed. *Handbook of Amyotrophic Lateral Sclerosis*. New York: Marcel Dekker, pp. 3–38.

Pantke, K.H., & Birbaumer, N. (2012). Die lebensqualität schwerstbetroffener nach einem schlaganfall mit locked-in syndrom. *Logos Interdisziplinär*, 20, 296–300.

Pfurtscheller, G., & Aranibar, A. (1979). Evaluation of event-related desynchronization (ERD) preceding and following self-paced movements. "*Electroencephalogr Clin Neurophysiol*, 46(2), 138–146.

Pfurtscheller, G., Mueller, G. R., Pfurtscheller, J., Gerner, H. J., & Rupp, R. (2003). "Thought"-control of functional electric stimulation to restore hand grasp in a patient with tetraplegia. *Neuroscience Letters*, 351(1), 169–174.

Ramos Murguialday, A., Hill, J., Bensch, M., Martens, S., Halder, S., Nijboer, F. Schoelkopf, B., Birbaumer, N., & Gharabaghi, A. (2011). Transition from the locked into the completely locked-in state: a physiological analysis. *Clin Neurophysiol*, 122(5), 925–933.

Razran, G. (1939). A simple technique for controlling subjective attitudes in salivary conditioning of adult human subjects. *Science*, 89, 160–161.

Razran, G. (1949a). Some psychological factors in the generalization of salivary conditioning to verbal stimuli. *The American Journal of Psychology*, 62(2), 247–256.

Razran, G. (1949b). Sentential and prepositional generalizations of salivary conditioning to verbal stimuli. *Science*, 109, 447–448.

Razran, G. (1961). The observable unconscious and the inferable conscious in current Soviet psychophysiology: interoceptive conditioning, semantic conditioning, and the orienting reflex. *Psychol Rev*, 68(2), 1–147.

Riehle, A., & Vaadia, E., Eds. (2005). *Motor Cortex in Voluntary Movements: A Distributed System for Distributed Functions*. Boca Raton: CRC Press.

Rockstroh, B., Elbert, T., Birbaumer, N., & Lutzenberger, W. (1989). *Slow Brain Potentials and Behavior* (2nd ed.). Baltimore: Urban & Schwarzenberg.

Ruf, C., De Massari, D., Wagner-Podmaniczky, F., Matuz, T., & Birbaumer, N. (2013). Semantic conditioning of salivary pH for communication. *Special Issues, Artificial Int. & Medicine*, 59(2), 91–98.

Ruiz, S., Lee, S., Soekadar, S. R., Caria, A., Veit, R., Kircher, T., Birbaumer, N., & Sitaram, R. (2013). Acquired self-control of insula cortex modulates emotion recognition and brain network connectivity in schizophrenia. *Hum Brain Mapp*, 34(1), 200–212.

Sellers, E. W., & Donchin, E. (2006). A P300-based brain-computer interface: initial tests by ALS patients. *Clin Neurophysiol*, 117(3), 538–548.

Silvoni, S., Cavinato, M., Volpato, C., Ruf, C., Birbaumer, N., & Piccione, F. (2013). Amyotrophic lateral sclerosis progression and stability of brain-computer interface communication. *Amyotroph Lateral Scler Frontotemporal Degener*, 14(5), 390–396.

Sitaram, R., Caria, A., Veit, R., Gaber, T., Rota, G., Kübler, A., Birbaumer, N. (2007a). FMRI brain-computer interface: a tool for neuroscientific research and treatment. *Computational Intelligence and Neuroscience*, 10, 1155–1165.

Sitaram, R., Zhang, H., Guan, C., Thulasidas, M., Hoshi, Y., Ishikawa, A., Shimizu, K., & Birbaumer N. (2007b). Temporal classification of multi-channel near infrared spectroscopy signals of motor imagery for developing a brain-computer interface. *NeuroImage*, 34(4), 1416–1427.

Strangman, G., Boas, D. A., & Sutton, J. P. (2002). Non-invasive neuroimaging using near-infrared light. *Biol Psychiatry*, 52(7), 679–693.

Swash, M., & Ingram, D. A. (1988). Preclinical and subclinical events in motor neuron disease. *J Neurol Neurosurg Psychiatry*, 51(2), 165–168.

Velliste, M., Perel, S., Spalding, M. C., Whitford, A. S., & Schwartz, A. B. (2008). Cortical control of a prosthetic arm for self-feeding. *Nature*, 453, 1098–1101.

Vlek, R. J., Steines, D., Szibbo, D., Kübler, A., Schneider, M. J., Haselager, P., Nijboer, F. (2012). Ethical issues in brain-computer interface research, development, and dissemination. *J Neurol Phys Ther*, 36(2), 94–99.

Volpato, C., Piccione, F., Silvoni, S., Cavinato, M., Palmieri, A., Meneghello, F., & Birbaumer, N. (2010). Working memory in amyotrophic lateral sclerosis: auditory event-related potentials and neuropsychological evidence. *J Clinical Neurophysiology*, 27(3), 198–206.

Wilhelm, B., Jordan, M., & Birbaumer, N. (2006). Communication in locked-in syndrome: effects of imagery on salivary pH. *Neurology*, 67(3), 534–535.

Wohlfart, S., & Wohlfart, G. (1935). Mikroskopie untersuchungen an progressive Muskel-atrophien. *Acta Med Scand (Suppl)*, 63, 1–137.

Wolpaw, J.R., Birbaumer, N., McFarland, D., Pfurtscheller, G., & Vaughan, T. (2002). Brain-computer interfaces for communication and control. *Clinical Neurophysiology*, 113(6), 767–791.

Wolpaw, J.R., & McFarland, D.J. (2004). Control of a two-dimensional movement signal by a noninvasive brain-computer interface in humans. *Proc Natl Acad Sci USA*, 101(51), 17849–17854.

7 Disorders of consciousness in an evolving neuroscience context

Graham Wilson[1] *and Eric Racine*[2]

Abbreviations

DOC	disorders of consciousness
DTI	diffusion tensor imaging
EEG	electroencephalography
EOL	end-of-life
fMRI	functional magnetic resonance imaging
MCS	minimally conscious state
PET	positron emission tomography
QOL	quality of life
VS/UWS	vegetative state/unresponsive wakefulness syndrome

Introduction

Patients with disorders of consciousness (DOC) pose medical, ethical, social, and scientific challenges. The past decades have yielded scientific advances that have kindled a better understanding of the complex mechanisms by which severe brain injury produces DOC (Racine, Rodrigue, et al., 2010). Moreover, these clinical innovations herald a paradigm shift in how physicians assess awareness and have led to improvements in prognostic practices and to the reevaluation of diagnostic classifications (Jox, Bernat, et al., 2012, Fins et al., 2008).

Despite this received knowledge, our understanding of DOC remains incomplete and is still evolving (Shiel et al., 2004). Advances in neuroscience research continue to challenge our traditional understandings of DOC, notably regarding whether these patients retain the ability to process pain stimuli or language (Coleman et al., 2007; Boly et al., 2008; Owen and Coleman, 2008). These developments have led us to question what an accurate understanding of a DOC really is (Fins et al., 2008). Do these advances give us access into the "thought processes" of these patients? Are we gaining better insights into their chances of recovery? If they have sufficient cognitive capabilities, could we communicate with them to learn about their end-of-life (EOL) preferences? Such questions are generated through novel techniques like neuroimaging, whose capabilities and limitations are yet to be established. Simultaneously, this novel information is being sought out by families and other stakeholders, particularly through the Internet and other media. The availability of this information, combined with the evolving landscape of medical knowledge, creates an environment that impacts the value of expertise and the nature of decision-making challenging the fundamental moral, legal, and social questions concerning DOC (Jox, Bernat, et al., 2012).

In this chapter, we present several of the ethical and social challenges that arise during the care and treatment of patients with DOC and consider how these impact both health-care professionals and the public. We review recent developments in neuroscience research on DOC and examine how these interact with the longstanding ethical challenges associated with these conditions.

Diagnosis and prognosis: the need for professional and public education

DOC are conditions that result from severe traumatic or nontraumatic brain injury and comprise coma, unresponsive wakefulness syndrome (UWS, formerly known as the vegetative state, or VS [Laureys et al., 2010]), and the minimally conscious state (MCS). Diagnosis and prognosis of DOC present both medical and ethical challenges. Differentiating these disorders and related conditions (e.g., locked-in syndrome) can be difficult, even with the assistance of supplementary tools like functional magnetic resonance imaging (fMRI) and electroencephalography (EEG; Brukamp, 2012, see also Chapter 5).

The current classification of DOC is based on clinical observation and interpretation of symptoms (Laureys, Owen, & Schiff, 2004). Yet criticism still persists that such clear-cut distinctions and criteria cannot be employed in clinical practice and medical terminology (Gosseries et al., 2004).

The "gold standard" for establishing whether a patient is aware or not is to study their activity and behavior (Plum & Posner, 1983) with consecutive neurobehavioral assessments at the bedside (Laureys et al., 2005) over a number of days and weeks, and at different times of the day (Gaccino et al., 1997; Andrews, 1996; Laureys, 2007). Only after a careful assessment of a patient's level of awareness and responsiveness is the diagnosis of coma, VS/UWS, or MCS possible. However, several sources of errors always exist. For example, behavioral assessment is not immune from subjectivity. Classifying signs of awareness is challenging because of fluctuating levels of arousal and deficits in attention, perception, and motor function (Chwala-Schlegel & Schabus, 2012). The subtle behavioral signs of consciousness and the irregularity of behaviors, whether meaningful or ambiguous, often lead to misinterpretations. Moreover, the prevalence of cases of DOC is low. Estimates of VS/UWS have been projected at 19 cases per million in a large European city (Powner, Hernandez, & Rives, 2004). As a result, physicians in many practice settings may have little experience with patients in this diagnostic category and are therefore unable to develop the necessary skills for accurate observation or the proper use of assessment tools (Majerus et al., 2005). Consequently, studies that have investigated the rate of misdiagnoses have suggested significant diagnostic inaccuracies (around 40%) (Childs, Mercer, & Childs, 1993; Andrews et al., 1996; Schnakers et al., 2009; McCann et al., 2012). For more details on this point, we invite readers to consult Chapters 1 and 4. Nevertheless, lower inaccuracy rates have been recently reported (Kuehlmeyer, Racine, Palmour et al., 2012; Kuehlmeyer et al., 2014). In a study targeting neurologists and utilizing case vignettes, a misdiagnosis rate of 7% for VS/UWS and 20% for MCS was observed. Interestingly, although a significantly higher confidence rate was found in neurologists who correctly diagnosed the patient than in those who erred, in this study the latter still had a relatively high level of confidence in their diagnostic skills. This finding may be problematic if it is generalized to the health-care profession, for it is unlikely this group will seek second opinions or further training (Kuehlmeyer, Racine, Palmour et al., 2012).

The causes of confusion and misdiagnosis remain unclear, but Gill-Thwaites has suggested a series of factors that could be involved, such as: (1) differential diagnosis and definitions (e.g., persistent and permanent vegetative state versus VS/UWS versus hyporesponsive, reflexive responsive, localizing responsive, and transitional state); (2) the assessor's previous knowledge and the lack of general health-care education about DOC; (3) the availability for frequent assessment of the patient over time; (4) the tool used to support the diagnosis; (5) inconsistent involvement of family members and caregivers as well as variability in the patient's medical and physical management (Gill-Thwaites, 2006).

Diagnostic inaccuracy also could result from the confusion over DOC in the medical community. For example, one study conducted by Youngner and colleagues found that health-care providers, including physicians involved in decision-making as well as staff involved in care but less in decision-making, such as nurses and residents, conflate persistent VS/UWS with brain death (Youngner et al., 1989). Such confusion has been found even among neurologists and neurosurgeons (Tomlinson, 1990) and has been previously discussed in the Canadian context (Young, Blume, & Lynch, 1989).

It appears that previous research and common neurological perspectives on DOC do not appear to have fully penetrated general health-care knowledge and practice (Racine, Rodrigue, et al., 2010). For instance, an investigation by Kuehlmeyer, Racine, Palmour et al. (2012) found that while several neurologists agreed that VS/UWS patients were not aware, a large proportion of them indicated that these patients were able to experience hunger and thirst, have emotions and thoughts, and perceive various somatosensory stimuli (like pain). This study also found that the most common error was to overestimate the patient as being in a MCS instead of VS/UWS.

The consequences of misdiagnoses can range from positive to detrimental. Misdiagnosis can have effects on the ongoing care of the patient by biasing prognostication and therapeutic strategy. It may lead to insufficient stimulation or inappropriate discharge locations. In some countries and jurisdictions, the diagnosis can influence EOL decisions and consideration for discontinuation of life-sustaining treatment, including artificial nutrition and hydration (McCann et al., 2012; Spinney, 2004; Demertzi et al., 2011). For the family or surrogate decision-makers, a misdiagnosis can lead to undue stress if questions are raised regarding the accuracy of the diagnosis (McCann et al., 2012). False-positives may cause the family to develop unrealistic expectations for recovery, communication, or other outcomes, and they may lead to expenses for futile treatments.

The challenge of clinical diagnosis clearly indicates the need for education and dissemination of more precise clinical scales (Racine, Rodrigue, et al., 2010). New tools (e.g., Coma Recovery Scale-Revised) have been developed and refined to address the limitations of the commonly used but crude Glasgow Coma Scale (Giacino, Kalmar, & Whyte, 2004). However, common to both the new and older tools are the ongoing challenges such as the subjective interpretation of the patient's behavior by the assessor and, in the case of the simple and well-known Glasgow Coma Scale, variability in application, especially across subspecialties (Crossman et al., 1998; Buechler et al., 1998).

Clinicians also appear to experience discomfort and distress during the diagnosis, prognosis, and care of patients with DOC. Studies have revealed how assessing levels of awareness and caring for these patients can lead to fear, confusion, self-doubt, and widely diverging views about the appropriate medical and ethical care of these patients (Montagnino & Ethier, 2007; Bell, 1986; McCann et al., 2012; Payne, Taylor, Stocking, & Sachs, 1996; Wilson et al., 2007). These studies have shown that health-care providers struggle with prognosis (and the uncertainty about patient outcome), a task essential for communication with families and decision-making about life-sustaining treatment or EOL care (Rodrigue et al., 2013).

The extent of this confusion is exemplified in a study from Racine et al. (2007) that used two American academic medical centers to conduct interviews with intensivists and neurointensivists. The 18 participating physicians first read a clinical vignette featuring a 40-year-old comatose male suffering from post-anoxic brain injury. Following cardiac arrest and resuscitation, the patient was still comatose a week later and over-breathing his ventilator. His pupils were reactive but his eyes did not follow any commands; he had no corneal, cough, or gag reflexes; and he withdrew to pain in response to noxious stimuli. Participants provided demographic information in addition to a prognosis and a prediction of outcome (Racine et al., 2007).

Physicians differed considerably in their predictions, with two main sources of prognostic variability emerging. First, a spectrum of responses was given in predicting long-term functional outcomes (e.g., responses ranged from fair/good to poor). Second, they revealed variation in their individual confidence levels of those reported outcomes (e.g., uncertain – certain). When these variations were categorized into prognostic quadrants, a majority of physicians fell into "those who believed the prognosis was poor but were uncertain." Significant variability was also observed in the type and degree of predicted outcomes when asked about cognitive, motor, and social deficits. For instance, while some physicians thought the patient would be free of motor problems (e.g., "I think he would have no motor problem[s]"), others anticipated permanent motor impairments (e.g., ". . . it'd be very unlikely that he would be able to sit up independently and move extremities in a purposeful fashion. I think it even less likely he'd be able to walk"; Racine et al., 2007).

Despite the need for more quantitative data, this study revealed an inconsistency among physicians that illustrates a real and substantive issue in health-care systems (Racine et al., 2007). Such variability among health-care teams could have substantial ethical and medical consequences in the care of patients with DOC if family members are receiving similar, wide-ranging, opinions about prognoses, potential recovery, and levels of certainty (Racine, 2013). We acknowledge that variability in opinions is inescapable because each health-care professional brings with them unique values, personalities, training, and experiences (Racine et al., 2007). Moreover, variability in clinical styles and philosophies, especially among physicians, is easy to conceive in clinical environments that require staff rotations. This is exemplified by a health-care professional who was reported stating, "[R]otations have to occur. And so yes, you do have different mindsets from different . . . physicians and different teams" (Rodrigue et al., 2011). Yet some sources of variability are subject to improvement. For example, a shared and concerted approach to patient care and communication with families may provide more time for discussion between members of the health-care team to ensure the best standards of practice are employed (Jeffery, 2005). Given the pluralistic nature of our contemporary societies and the challenges of conveying diagnostic and prognostic information in such complex social and religious contexts, it is important to acknowledge such "biases" and keep our health-care professionals updated about them. By being aware of their existence, providers can consciously act on them and offer more coherent messages to family members and the public (Racine et al., 2009).

The reality that health-care professionals seem unaware of, or do not acknowledge, these biases and potential influences merits further attention and continued educational efforts from the medical and ethics communities. If physicians do not perceive these influences, they may lure themselves into thinking they are providing objective and unbiased prognoses. Acknowledging these subjective biases could help achieve a more socially aware and objective ethical-clinical perspective (Racine, 2013).

The need for professional education is reflective of an equally pressing need for broader public education. Studies find a sizeable gap between current expert medical views and public views and also find that the distinct states of brain death, VS/UWS, and coma are not well distinguished by the public (Shanteau & Linin, 1990; Siminofff, Burant, & Youngner, 2004). A principal reason for this confusion is the lack of availability of quality information (Fins et al., 2008). For example, in a study of 30 motion pictures created between 1970 and 2004, Wijdicks and collaborators found that coma was usually incorrectly described and misinterpreted. Most (18 out of 30) motion pictures depicted patients who woke up suddenly, even from prolonged coma, with intact cognition. The authors found that "all actors except one remained well groomed with normal muscular, tanned appearance," and none of the coma actors displayed contractures or were tracheotomized. Only two out of the 30 motion pictures (*Dream*

Life of Angels and *Reversal of Fortune*) provided a reasonably accurate depiction of coma (Wijdicks & Wijdicks, 2006). Definitional difficulties in distinguishing neurological disorders have also been found in the depiction of coma (2001–2005) in American newspapers (Wijdicks & Wijdicks, 2005). The use of such technical jargon in chronic DOC may lead to poor knowledge transfer and misunderstandings in the public (Racine, Rodrigue, et al., 2010).

Similarly, examining media coverage of VS/UWS in the Terri Schiavo case, a study from Racine et al. (2008) found important mischaracterizations of this patient's prognosis and behavioral repertoire (e.g., she responds, she reacts), which were clearly inconsistent with her diagnosis of VS/UWS. One fifth of the 1,141 articles examined contained statements to the effect that she might recover after many years in the VS/UWS. This result is consistent with evidence from another study that suggests that more than one-fifth of families of brain-dead patients believe those individuals will still recover (Siminoff, Mercer, & Arnold, 2003). Furthermore, several strong expressions were used to describe withdrawal of life-support (e.g., murder, euthanasia). Out of all the news reports and editorials published about this case between 1990 and 2005, less than 1% of the articles explained the clinical features of DOC to the public (e.g., coma, VS/UWS, MCS, or brain death) (Racine et al., 2008; Racine, Rodrigue, et al., 2010).

These examples emphasize the gap between expert perspectives and the public understanding of DOC. Such misunderstandings and misconceptions can confuse families of patients and the lay public about the diagnosis, prognosis, and behavioral repertoire of patients in states of disordered consciousness (Macdonald et al., 2008). This kind of misunderstanding can fuel mistrust during the interactions of the medical team with the family and lead to difficulties in communication of poor prognosis as identified by Bernat (2006) and Fins (2005b). Ethical and cultural barriers based on traditions, beliefs about critical illness, and disagreements due to misunderstandings can all contribute to variability and confusion about DOC (Bernat, 2004; Racine, 2010). As a result of all of these factors, both health-care professionals and the public remain unclear about these conditions. Further, the sizeable challenges posed by diagnoses, general health-care providers' common misunderstanding of DOC, variability in the use of common clinical scales and tools, and developing specialized literature, all suggest a stronger role for expert teams of neurologists, critical care physicians, medical ethicists, and other specialists (Andrews et al., 1996).

New controversies about life–sustaining therapy, quality of life, and end–of–life care

VS/UWS and MCS patients require various levels of medical support to stay alive because of their preserved brainstem and autonomic functions. Sometimes, the only treatment needed is artificial hydration and nutrition because of the incapacity of patients to swallow (Lennard-Jones, 2000). In the hope of recovery, patients can be supported over months and even years, but over time chances of recovery diminish. The care of such chronically unconscious patients raises vexing medical, ethical, and social questions concerning quality of life (QOL), EOL care, and life-sustaining treatment.

Intense ethical and societal debates arise regarding the ethical justification of administering life-sustaining treatment in these patients, particularly with regard to the use of artificial hydration and nutrition. Few legal and ethical guidelines exist regarding EOL treatment in patients with DOC. The Canadian Medical Association, the American Academy of Neurology, and several other medical organizations have opined that artificial nutrition and hydration should be considered a treatment, like other medical treatments, for which a proxy decision-maker can consent or refuse (Bacon, Williams, & Gordon, 2007; American Academy of Neurology, 1989). For example, the code of ethics of the Canadian Medical Association specifies that physicians should "ascertain wherever possible and recognize [the] patient's wishes about the initiation, continuation or cessation of life-sustaining treatment" (Canadian Medical Association, 2004). Accordingly, once a diagnosis and a prognosis are reliably confirmed, and the previous wishes of the patient are known, patients can be treated aggressively or life-sustaining therapy can be withheld or withdrawn to allow the patient to die if this would have been their wish (Bernat, 2006). These discussions raise critical questions about what evidence and standard of proof is needed when decisions are being made about the fates of those who cannot communicate their wishes (Bruno et al., 2013).

In Canada and the United States, the medical, legal, and ethical consensuses regarding withdrawal or withholding of life support were developed based on precedent-setting medicolegal cases of patients with DOC, especially Karen Quinlan and Nancy Cruzan (Pence, 2004). However, recent public debates and some religious groups, notably in the United States and Italy, have called into question past expert medical, scientific, legal, and ethical consensuses. This trend was visible in the Schiavo case where large-scale political and legal activities were sparked by debates over the removal of her feeding tube in the United States (Perry, Churchill, & Kirshner, 2005). Similarly, in Italy, the case of Eluana Englaro, who was in a chronic state of VS/UWS, has provoked passionate debates and the involvement of courts and pro-life groups as well as reactions from the Catholic Church.

Pope John Paul II issued an opinion in 2004 that appeared to contradict the previous Roman Catholic doctrinal acceptance of withdrawal of life-support. In a joint statement of the World Federation of Catholic Medical Associations and the Pontifical Academy for Life, presented at the International Congress on "Life sustaining treatments and vegetative state: Scientific advances and ethical dilemmas," withdrawal of life-support was equated to euthanasia and therefore condemned:

> [t]he possible decision of withdrawing nutrition and hydration, necessarily administered to VS/UWS patients in an assisted way, is followed inevitably by the patients' death as a direct consequence. Therefore, it has to be considered a genuine act of euthanasia by omission, which is morally unacceptable.

(Pontifical Academy for Life and the World Federation of Catholic Medical Associations, 2004)

In his address to the participants of this congress, the Pope declared that:

> [t]he administration of water and food, even when provided by artificial means, always represents a natural means of preserving life, not a medical act. Its use, furthermore, should be considered, in principle, ordinary and proportionate, and as such morally obligatory, insofar as and until it is seen to have attained its proper finality, which in the present case consists in providing nourishment to the patient and alleviation of his suffering. . . . The evaluation of probabilities, founded on waning hopes for recovery when the vegetative state is prolonged beyond a year, cannot ethically justify the cessation or interruption of minimal care for the patient, including nutrition and hydration. (John Paul II, 2004)

This strong endorsement of the sanctity of life and public reactions to the Schiavo case triggered some American states to reexamine legislation allowing proxy decision-makers to withdraw artificial hydration and nutrition from unconscious patients without formal advance directives. In the past few years, some advocacy groups have become more vocal and, consequently, withdrawal of life-support remains a source of discord in the public domain. In response to conservative positions, the American Academy of Neurology has reiterated its position regarding the acceptability of withdrawal of life-support based on the three standards (pure autonomy, substituted judgment, and best interests) (Bacon et al., 2007).

Differences in societal and medical practice, specifically contextual (e.g., use of time, resource allocation, public understanding of DOC) and relational (e.g., relationship to the patient, disagreements with decision-making, family's interests, etc.) can shape how decisions about life-sustaining treatment are made (Ganz et al., 2006; Rodrigue et al., 2013). Surveys of physicians' attitudes towards withdrawal of artificial nutrition and hydration and decisions about EOL care have shown considerable diversity among different health professions and countries (Rodrigue et al., 2011; Kuehlmeyer et al., 2012; Kuehlmeyer et al., 2014; Demertzi et al., 2013; Demertzi et al., 2011; Lanzerath & Feeser, 1998; Grubb et al., 1996; Hurst et al., 2007; Payne, 1996). For instance, one study comparing Canadian and German perspectives of VS/UWS found that more Canadian participants favored the cessation of life-sustaining treatment – an outcome which might be explained by the more rationalistic and utilitarian approach taken in Canada versus the deontological philosophical traditions upheld in Germany (Kuelmeyer et al., 2014). Moreover, Canadian participants viewed time, resource allocation (Rodrigue et al., 2013), and long-term care placement as the most ethically challenging issues, a perception not held by their German counterparts. One hypothesis is that physicians in the German health-care system have greater access to long-term care facilities, nursing homes for patients who require artificial respiration, and specialized centers for patients with DOC (Huber & Kuehlmeyer, 2012). Variability in opinions was also observed in a study from the United States, in which only a quarter of hemato-oncologists and more than 40% of other respondents (e.g., nurses and other specialists) answered "yes" to the question of whether artificial nutrition should always be kept (Wilkinson et al., 2009). This diversity of practices surrounding EOL care is even seen between teams working within an integrated health network (Rodrigue et al., 2011), thus exemplifying the influence which legal regulations, institutional medical practice, and health-care systems may have implicitly on health-care providers.

The question of a patient's QOL also surfaces in discussions and decisions about whether to withhold or withdraw life-sustaining treatments for patients with poor prognoses. Research into the QOL for patients with VS/UWS or MCS is limited, since by definition these patients are unable to communicate. Nevertheless, qualitative estimations have been inferred from health-care professionals. For example, a study by Jennett (1976) reported that nearly 90% of physicians regarded VS/UWS as worse than death. A more recent European survey found similar results, particularly when professionals looked from the perspective of the family, again identifying chronic VS/UWS as worse than death (Demertzi et al., 2011). Alternatively, several studies have reported that despite being socially isolated or having difficulties in daily activities, patients with severe disabilities experience a good QOL (Post et al., 1998; Albrecht & Devlieger, 1999; Bruno et al., 2013).

Views on the moral relevance and practical utility of "QOL" in medical and ethical discussions vary greatly. Many scholars have emphasized the risks of speculating about a patient's QOL given the subjective nature of assessing what is a good life and a life "worth living" (Sim, 1997; Phipps & Whyte, 1999; Racine et al., 2007; Kuehlmeyer, Borasio & Jox, 2012). For example, as quoted by one physician:

> [i]t depends on the patient . . . I can only comment on functional status. It seems like it's the patient's job to interpret what functional status means to them in terms of their quality of life. So, quality of life is inherently value laden, and it's only for the patient to decide for a particular functional status what the quality associated with that is. (Racine et al., 2007)

Other criticisms of using QOL in medical practice stem from the findings that health-care professionals tend to underestimate a patient's QOL (Miller & Fins, 2006). Moreover, physicians' and patients' perception of QOL may change over time (e.g., patients adapting to chronic disabilities through homeostatic processes of well-being) (Nizzi et al., 2012). Consequently, some have attempted to distinguish between the "objective" and "subjective" factors in assessing QOL (Phipps & Whyte, 1999). In this scheme, objective factors include social support, employment, and the ability to communicate with others, while subjective factors are defined by the patient him or herself (Phipps & Whyte, 1999).

Despite the controversies surrounding QOL, the beneficial effects of treatments need to be assessed by clinicians. Efforts should be made to disentangle the medical goals of treatments (and outcomes) from the more subjective assessment of these goals and outcomes in order to avoid providers (and family members) imposing or projecting personal views on a patient. The concept of shared decision-making captures this collaborative approach in which the expertise and experience of providers and family members join forces to reach respectful and mutually acceptable decisions (Racine & Shevell, 2009).

DOC represents a difficult group, ethically, for surrogate decision-makers. Disagreements and conflicts often arise because of the religious beliefs of the family, diverging views on QOL, miscommunications, refusal of interventions by physicians, and more. Families often report struggling with the role as proxies when making decisions according to the patient's wishes or if the patient's best interests are in conflict with their own personal views (Rodrigue et al., 2013). For example, "Should we continue the patient's treatment at all costs? Should we treat cardiac arrest or kidney failure or pneumonia in these patients?" (Bruno et al., 2013). The fear of being responsible for the death of the patient was a major factor preventing family members from making a decision and they would rather ". . . let an external event or factor such as fate, the disease or the patient himself decide" (Kuehlmeyer, Borasio, & Jox, 2012).

The medical community needs to reach a better agreement about the care of patients with DOC, to ensure more effective communication as advocated by Jox et al. (2012). Since families of patients with DOC may encounter physicians who take different approaches to QOL and EOL decision-making, physicians must acknowledge this variability to ensure their responses do not incorporate their own subjective perspective. For example, characteristics such as age, religious beliefs, experience, specialty and subspecialty, and practice setting have all been shown to influence EOL care in the intensive care setting (Cook et al., 1995; Randolph et al., 1997; Keenan et al., 1998; Prendergast et al., 1998; Asch et al., 1999; Marcin et al., 1999; Rebagliato et al., 2000; Rocker et al., 2006). As previously noted, one European study showed drastically different approaches to EOL practices in the intensive care unit between southern Europe (Greece, Turkey, Spain, Portugal, Italy), northern Europe (the United Kingdom, Finland, Ireland, Denmark, Sweden, Netherlands) and Central Europe (Belgium, Czech Republic, Germany, Austria, Switzerland). They discovered that physicians from northern Europe were more likely to withhold or withdraw life-support than were physicians in southern Europe (Sprung et al., 2003; Ganz et al., 2006).

The controversies around clinical management of patients with DOC are personified by the discrepancy between how a physician or nurse would treat himself or herself versus a patient (Gillick et al., 1993). When asked to imagine themselves in a chronic VS/UWS, most clinicians agreed (66%) to withdraw treatment and did not want to be kept alive (82%), but in chronic MCS fewer agreed to withdraw treatment (28%), and wished not to be kept alive (33%) (Demertzi et al., 2011). It is important that physicians acknowledge these biases to ensure they do not unduly impact the EOL experience of the patient and the subsequent bereavement process for the family (Jeffery, 2005).

To ensure incorporation of new evidence-based advances, attention should be paid to the real-world practices and challenges experienced by professionals in diagnosis, prognosis, life-sustaining treatment, and EOL care – especially given that DOC are such complex conditions (Rodrigue et al., 2013). It is important that health-care providers recognize how social and contextual factors, as well as disparities in the public understanding, can shape clinical encounters and the decision-making process. This pattern of neglect will remain unattended unless a greater commitment is given to empirical research to deepen health-care professionals' self-awareness when formulating impartial clinical recommendations (Racine, Rodrigue, et al., 2010).

Disorders of consciousness in an evolving neuroscience context

Current debates about advances in understanding DOC have surfaced, particularly regarding advances in functional neuroimaging and improving diagnostic and prognostic accuracy (Fins et al., 2008; Gofton et al., 2009). Despite the publication of provocative case reports, there is no "magic bullet" test that can sensitively and specifically determine the presence of consciousness. The elicitation of clinical signs remains the diagnostic standard. However, the accurate evaluation of cognitive function by observing behavioral signs to determine awareness is difficult. For instance, patients emerging from unconsciousness may lack the capacity to perform voluntary movements; their arousal and awareness levels are subjective to fluctuations; and their actions are vulnerable to misinterpretation. Moreover, the selection of reliable and validated assessment tools is influenced by financial restrictions, the expertise of the team members, and whether the assessment is occurring at the acute or chronic stages (McCann et al., 2012).

The findings that patients with VS/UWS are able to preserve certain cognitive functions have raised controversy both medically and ethically, particularly regarding whether clinical observations are truly assessing consciousness per se. The fact that patients with DOC may in fact be aware alters his or her legal and ethical standing, and potentially his or her therapeutic and social standing as well. These findings have sparked hope that far more can be done for, and learned from, these patients (Fins, 2005a).

One such revealing case is that of Terry Wallis, who suffered a traumatic brain injury in 1984, was diagnosed with VS/UWS, and was refused further examination until 2003, when he awoke and started to speak (Fins & Schiff, 2006). Even after extended periods of time in a disordered consciousness (e.g., three months post-onset for patients with nontraumatic brain injury and more than one year for patients with traumatic brain injury), patients have been reported to recover, bringing into question the diagnostic and prognostic guidelines used at the bedside (Luaute et al., 2010; Estraneo et al., 2010; Kuehlmeyer et al., 2013).

New technological developments like diffusion tensor imaging (DTI), fMRI, positron emission tomography (PET), and EEG are promising tools of the future. The ability of these developments to permit the measurement of brain function in both the active and resting states of patients who do not have muscle function has generated both excitement and controversy. In this section, we will analyze these issues and describe the type of research being conducted internationally.

Neuroimaging in VS/UWS and MSC

Since the late 1990s, several studies have used and employed neuroimaging in VS/UWS and MCS. Some of the early results questioned common assumptions about the VS/UWS (Fins et al., 2008). For example, in a comparative study of severely brain-injured MCS and VS/UWS patients, Coleman and colleagues found that three out of seven VS/UWS patients and two out of five MCS patients showed "significant temporal lobe responses in the low-level auditory contrast" (Coleman et al., 2007) in a task involving a contrast between auditory stimuli and a silence baseline. The authors concluded that "these results provide further evidence that some vegetative patients retain islands of preserved cognitive function and that in the absence of behavioral evidence, functional imaging provides a valuable tool for the assessment team" (Coleman et al., 2007).

The most discussed report in this regard was published in 2006 by Adrian Owen and colleagues, who examined the brain functions of a 23-year-old woman who suffered a severe traumatic brain injury (Owen et al., 2006). The clinical diagnosis of VS/UWS was established. Owen and colleagues then gave her mental imagery tasks, such as imagining playing tennis and navigating around her house. Owen and colleagues found that her fMRI brain activation patterns were similar in location to those of normal subjects performing the mental imagery tasks (Owen et al., 2006). They concluded that "these results confirm that, despite fulfilling the clinical criteria for a diagnosis of VS/UWS, this patient retained the ability to understand spoken commands and to respond to them through her brain activity, rather than through speech or movement." The authors also asserted that the patient made a "decision to cooperate with the authors," which "confirmed beyond any doubt that she was consciously aware of herself and her surroundings" (Owen et al., 2006, Owen & Coleman, 2008).

Such advancement in neuroimaging has an important ethical dimension. As noted by Fins (2010), the discovery that some behaviorally nonresponsive patients (as ascertained by standard clinical tests) "were not only conscious and responsive to their environment, but also able to process language and perhaps experience the profound isolation of being able to understand but not respond . . . [is] spine-chilling" (Fins, 2010). A misdiagnosis could prevent a patient from receiving the appropriate therapeutic intervention; the misdiagnosed patient may be transferred to unsuitable long-term care facilities or be deprived of social stimulation.

Accordingly, a larger clinical study was undertaken to better assess the proportion of VS/UWS and MCS patients who could communicate and to improve the reliability of fMRI-based communication methods. This study included 23 VS/UWS patients and 31 MCS patients with diverse etiologies. It clearly showed that some patients, specifically those with traumatic brain injuries, "were able to modulate their brain activity by generating voluntary, reliable, and repeatable blood-oxygenated-level-dependent responses" when they were prompted to conduct mental imagery tasks (Monti et al., 2010). For two of these five patients, further clinical examination was unable to identify reliable responsive behavior. These observations are important, for they suggest that a dissociation can occur between, on the one hand, best attempts to identify meaningful behavior through bedside examination and, on the other hand, fMRI-based detection of voluntary and specific response. Amazingly, it has been suggested that a consistent proportion of VS/UWS and MCS patients are able to communicate in this way, a finding that dramatically challenges the medical and ethical reliability of bedside diagnoses in DOC (Monti et al., 2010).

Monti et al. (2012) investigated this dissociation further. In this study, a patient with traumatic brain injury was described who showed no evidence of command-following during standard behavioral tests but who could produce distinctive responses in selected brain regions by "willfully" altering his brain activity. In this fMRI paradigm, the patient was asked, following a cue (e.g., tone), to change his attentional focus from a house to a face (or vice versa). This shift in attention was shown to produce a distinct change in activity from the parahippocampal gyrus to the fusiform gyrus or vice versa. Despite the stimulus remaining unchanged throughout the experiment, the cues prompted time-locked alterations of activity between these functionally predefined brain regions similar to that of healthy volunteers. This led one author to state that "this change is driven not by the external stimulus per se but rather by the will or the intention of the participant to focus on one or the other aspect of the stimulus and is therefore a reliable indicator of conscious intent" (Owen, 2013).

The reliability of bedside diagnoses has also been questioned through EEG research. In an attempt to detect evidence of command-following, Cruse et al. (2011) reported a new EEG technique that could decode specific mental imagery responses (e.g., wiggling all of the toes versus squeezing the right hand) in patients who met the criteria of VS/UWS. Using this approach, three of these patients (19%) were able to consistently produce the appropriate EEG responses when given a specific command (e.g., "wiggle your toes" or "squeeze your right hand") despite being behaviorally unresponsive. A follow-up study with 23 MCS patients found similar robust responses, with 23% of the patients demonstrating residual cognitive abilities (Cruse et al., 2012).

Caution should be taken with regards to negative results, for the absence of brain-activity modulation is not dispositive (Bardin et al., 2011). Fluctuation of arousal, cognitive dysfunction in memory, language, visual, or auditory processing, the latency of the response, or simply a failure in the imaging method itself (e.g., just because a statistical analysis shows no "significant" activity in a particular brain region does not necessarily mean there was no activity in that part of the brain) could all lead to an absent or inadequate patient response (Fins, 2010). These findings emphasize the need for better diagnostic guidelines and the incorporation of standardized neuroimaging procedures.

Contrary to neuroimaging research into VS/UWS, which has tended to question the integrity of bedside diagnoses, investigations into MCS through fMRI, PET, DTI, and more have tended to support the premise that MCS patients produce distinctive effects when compared to VS/UWS patients. In a study by Fernández-Espejo et al. (2011), researchers were able to employ DTI to distinguish 15 MCS patients from 10 VS/UWS by generating and differentiating the diffusivity maps of the subcortical white matter and thalamic regions. Not only did their DTI results predict each patient's scores on the Coma Recovery Scale-Revised, but they were also able to assign each patient to their appropriate diagnostic category with an accuracy rate of 95% (Fernández-Espejo et al., 2011). Accordingly, neuroimaging research has tended to complement behavioral diagnoses for MCS as well as uphold the distinction between VS/UWS and MCS. For example, perceptions of pain in MCS patients are similar to those observed in healthy participants when visualized through PET activation (e.g., activation of the "pain matrix" elicits activity in the anterior and frontoparietal cingulate cortices and the secondary somatosensory cortex; Boly et al., 2008, see Chapter 2). This is much different in patients diagnosed with VS/UWS; their responses are much weaker and limited to the primary somatosensory area and thalamus (Laureys et al., 2002; Boly et al., 2008). Brain activation patterns of VS/UWS patients to noxious stimuli are also isolated compared to the more integrated responses of MCS patients because of the preserved connectivity between primary and secondary areas of the cortex (Laureys et al., 2002; Boly et al., 2008).

Whether the differential diagnosis of VS/UWS and MCS is useful is debatable, though studies have shown this distinction can have therapeutic and ethical implications. For example, fMRI studies have shown that patients with MCS are more likely to have partially preserved networks involved in pain (Boly et al., 2008), language (Schiff et al., 2005), and emotion (Laureys et al., 2004), and may therefore benefit more from analgesic treatment or other interventions aimed to improve QOL (Boly et al., 2008; Chatelle et al., 2012). Better outcomes and chances of recovering higher levels of consciousness are thought to be more likely in MCS in comparison to patients diagnosed with VS/UWS (Luaute, 2010; Hirschberg, 2011). Moreover, several countries have developed legal regulations that do not allow the removal of life-sustaining treatment from patients in MCS but permit it in patients with VS/UWS (Ferreira, 2007; Perry et al., 2005; Gevers, 2005).

Information on a patient's prognosis can also be provided by functional neuroimaging. For example, as described by Di et al. (2007), only those patients with VS/UWS capable of activating the peri-sylvian cortical language regions of their brains would later go on to recover clinical signs of awareness. In a similar study by Owen et al. (2006), a patient with a traumatic brain injury showed clinical signs of awareness 11 months post-injury after generating "willful patterns" of brain activity despite being clinically diagnosed as VS/UWS. It is therefore not surprising that family members are interested in such imaging advances to learn more about the prognosis for survival, chances of good neurological functioning, or the recovery of awareness.

These applications of neuroimaging were taken a step further by Owen & Coleman (2008) and subsequently refined by Monti et al. (2010), who employed brain activity modulation to communicate "yes" and "no" responses. When they applied this technique in a traumatic brain injury patient diagnosed as VS/UWS, this patient was able to communicate biographical information such as his father's name and the last place he visited before he had his accident five years earlier (Monti et al., 2010). It was suggested by Owen (2013) that such applications could theoretically be employed by investigators to address such ethical issues as whether or not the patients were feeling pain. Legally, fMRI-based communication could permit patients to designate a lawyer or family member to take care of affairs that are too complex for simple yes/no communication. Similarly, developments in EEG-based brain computer interfaces are improving quickly and could be utilized by patients to improve their QOL by controlling their environment or expressing their thoughts (Cruse et al., 2011, 2012; Owen, 2013).

These examples illustrate the ethical and legal challenges that accompany these developments in neuroscience research. The obvious next question is whether or not patients with sufficient "residual cognitive capabilities" could use these techniques to communicate their EOL preferences, decisions about life-sustaining treatment, experimental therapies, and more. In terms of treatment planning, such choices are already suggested through fMRI (Sorger et al., 2012) and EEG methods (Lulé et al., 2013). Nevertheless, it is the task of the medical and ethical communities to determine whether such "yes" or "no" paradigms are sufficient to establish whether a patient is emotionally and cognitively capable of making such complex decisions. These neuroimaging developments have a significant potential to give patients with DOC more autonomy and improved QOL. Consequently, clinicians and other specialists should be prepared to respond to more requests from family members and surrogate decision-makers for novel diagnostic procedures (Jox, Bernat, et al., 2012).

As stated by some neurologists, these research techniques are still evolving and may not be ready for broad use and dissemination (Hopkin, 2006). Nevertheless, given these recent results, it is probable that advances in neuroscience will contribute to and expand our understanding of DOC and improve diagnosis and prognosis. There are a number of issues that need closer attention before such promise can be delivered beyond the use of such research tools. For example, one of the key challenges in fMRI research concerns the acquisition and interpretation of the data yielded by functional neuroimaging and, in particular, its ability to reveal signs of consciousness in response to simple tasks reliably (Racine & Bell, 2008). Moreover, several of the scientific challenges have ethical implications that should be investigated, such as validating current procedures on a larger number of patients, standardizing the methodological approaches to eliciting brain activation, and developing guidelines for the interpretation of brain activation in MCS and VS/UWS (Bernat & Rottenberg, 2007).

Although new technologies like fMRI cannot replace the clinical assessment at the bedside, these technologies may provide additive information about cognitive function or identify meaningful responses in patients where clinical examination did not. Research and treatment centers should start to trial these techniques as a means to validate challenging diagnoses or monitor accuracy. They can be used to help family or surrogate decision-makers understand the neurological status of the patient (Fins, 2010). Moreover, widely available technologies like EEG may lower institutional barriers like cost and permit more widespread adoption of these technologies in routine care (Cruse et al., 2011). For that reason, large prospective investigations should evaluate the clinical value of novel technologies (e.g., fMRI, EEG, PET) and identify which etiology of DOC, duration, and clinical presentation are best suited for this patient population. The cost-effectiveness of such technologies has not been established and may merit ethical justification due to the low prevalence of such disorders (Overgaard & Overgaard, 2011; Coleman et al., 2009; Racine, Rodrigue, et al., 2010). The ethical and social aspects of resource allocation will be discussed later in this chapter.

The diagnostic potential and basic insights generated by neuroimaging tools will likely also be refined with the use of multiple imaging modalities (Schiff et al., 2007). For example, the combination of techniques like MRI with magnetic resonance spectroscopy with DTI is an interesting development. Magnetic resonance spectroscopy allows quantifying chemical compounds or metabolites related to neuronal integrity and neuronal energetic function while DTI allows assessing the integrity of white matter. These techniques, or the combination of these techniques, could lead to more precise measures of the potential for brain-injury patients to recover and respond to treatments (Machado et al., 2009; Tshibanda et al., 2009; Yuan et al., 2007; Huisman, 2004; Voss et al., 2006).

How may the evolution of neuroimaging affect physicians, patients, and families as well as interactions with patients with disorders of consciousness?

The evolving field of neuroscience has generated excitement and enthusiasm in the scientific community and stakeholders (including the relatives of patients diagnosed with DOC). Because information is now so easily accessible to the public, physicians must be increasingly prepared to answer questions and requests for investigational technologies. Does fMRI or EEG improve the diagnostic accuracy of VS/UWS? Or MCS? Does PET give us better insights into a patient's chances of recovery? These questions, in addition to others about the potential use of neuroimaging in DOC, raise important ethical questions.

Despite the cautionary statements found in the original papers, controversial interpretations, and confusion about neuroimaging, research in VS/UWS and MCS has been observed in publically available information and the media (Jox, Bernat, et al., 2012; Racine, 2010). Investigations into how this information is presented to the public have found that functional imaging technologies are rarely explained in a comprehensive manner (Racine, Waldman, et al., 2010; Racine et al., 2006). As a result, family members and surrogate decision-makers may approach physicians with unrealistic expectations. Clinicians should therefore also be aware of these misunderstandings and be prepared to explain not only the principles behind neuroimaging but also the diagnostic uncertainty that may remain even after the test (Racine & Bell, 2008). Physicians should communicate their level of confidence or uncertainty about the patient's diagnosis and prognosis to promote trustful relationships with family members and surrogate decision-makers. By doing so they facilitate and support an informed autonomous decision-making process (Jox, Bernat, et al., 2012; Bernat, 2009).

Neuroimaging results may help surrogate decision-makers and families to comprehend the clinical realities and manage the limited prospects of recovery following a diagnosis. Further investigations are needed to understand how the detection of awareness in patients with DOC affects family members and surrogate decision-makers and their behaviors, relationships with health-care providers, and the decision-making process. For instance, if a patient is shown to be irreversibly unaware, do family members speak to and handle the patient differently than if they were shown to be aware (Jox, Bernat, et al., 2012)?

Supporting the informed consent process in clinical care and in research based on innovative neurotechnology

In clinical care

It is fundamental, for both ethical and legal reasons, to support the informed consent process and to ensure that medical decisions are consistent with previously expressed wishes. In the absence of such declarations, decision-making must be consistent with the best interests of the patient. However, because patients with DOC cannot communicate, they cannot participate directly in decision-making. If patients have written advance directives, these should be respected and should guide decisions, although state or local variability may impact the scope and application of advance directives (Canadian Medical Association, 1992; Singer, Robertson, & Roy, 1996; Godlovitch, Mitchell, & Doig, 2005). However, because many victims of traumatic brain injury are young and because the injuries result from unanticipated events, it is common for patients not to have documented preferences for life-sustaining treatment. In addition, the interpretation of advance directives is challenging because of their ambiguity and because of the discomfort of many health-care providers in making assumptions about subjective judgments concerning QOL (Thompson, Barbour, & Scwartz, 2003; Racine et al., 2009). In the absence of advance directives when the patient is incapacitated, decision-making authority is usually delegated to family members (Godlovitch, Mitchell, & Doig, 2005). When this occurs, there are three basic surrogate (proxy) decision-making models that respect the autonomy and preferences of a patient as well as the patient's well-being in absence of decision-making capacity. Ethics committees can provide advice in unclear cases and more formal mechanisms like the appointment of legal guardians may help resolve difficult cases where no agreement can be reached within families or between family members and the health-care team (Godlovitch et al., 2005).

In clinical research

The participation of patients with DOC in research protocols involving functional neuroimaging procedures, drugs, and neurostimulation also raises the vexing issue of patient or proxy consent and the consideration of the patient's preferences and best interests (Fins et al., 2008; Fins, 2005b; Miller and Fins, 2006). The potential volunteer previously might have written advance directives specifically for research participation (a research living will or research advance directive) to provide guidance on his or her prior wishes. These preferences might be to consent to participate in minimal-risk research only; to refuse to participate in research involving certain procedures; or to participate in research protocols with higher than minimal risk. In such cases where a directive exists, a pure autonomy standard (i.e., precedence of previously expressed judgments of the volunteer) should apply. In the much more common circumstance in which there are no specific directives for research participation, the volunteer may have designated, through a durable power of attorney, a proxy decision-maker (sometimes called a research agent) empowered to make research participation decisions. The decision would then lie in the hands of this formally designated research proxy decision-maker, based on the wishes of the volunteer and applicable legal provisions of the jurisdiction (Miller & Fins, 2006).

Most often, however, the potential volunteer will not have executed advance directives for research purposes or have formally designated through a durable power of attorney a proxy decision-maker for such decisions. In this more common scenario, practices vary depending on the circumstances and the applicable legal and regulatory context. An existing health-care power of attorney could serve as a research decision-maker. A legal guardian may be court-appointed as the legally authorized representative, or an informal decision-maker (typically from the volunteer's family) may give consent for research participation. Close collaboration with the institutional research ethics board responsible for the approval of the research protocol is strongly recommended beyond the initial approval of the protocol. Following any of these options, the proxy decision-maker should respect the previous wishes of the volunteer, and when clear wishes are unknown she should use the best interest standard (i.e., judge based on the values and prior wishes of the volunteer) to decide what is in the patient's best interests. During discussions with the family, any confusion between informed consent for care and informed consent for research should be clarified and addressed (Miller and Fins, 2006). However, the mere incapacity to consent should not systematically exclude these patients from research. Research participation can be justified and ethical if consent by proxy is obtained (and a proper proxy decision-making mechanism identified) and approval by a research ethics board is granted (Fins, 2008).

Common to the context of proxy decision-making in the clinical and research context is the underlying need for more people to put advanced directives in place. In addition, the specificity of directives could be enhanced. For example, boilerplate advance directive forms could feature various clinical and research scenarios to simplify decisions for patients (and families). While these measures would help, they would not solve all issues or replace sensitive clinical approaches. Finally, a challenging scenario is likely to surface if greater confidence is acquired in the capacity to establish forms of communication with patients diagnosed as being behaviorally in VS/UWS and MCS, as reported in recent functional neuroimaging studies (Monti, 2010). What would be the clinical and technical criteria to establish the capacity of these patients to communicate reliably their preferences for research participation or clinical care through modalities like fMRI or EEG when they remain largely unresponsive?

Resource allocation

Today's public health-care systems are constrained by limited resources and are challenged to uphold a level of care that is incompatible with the growing demand for health care and novel technologies. This deficit makes it almost impossible to fulfill all claims for resources. Although some patients with DOC require minimally invasive care, the services required may consume considerable human and financial resources (Zeman, 1997). In 1994, the Multi-Society Task Force estimated that the total annual cost of adults and children in a VS/UWS, in the United States, was between $1 and $7 billion (Multi-Society Task Force, 1994). It can be assumed that, 20 years later, costs have increased substantially.

Health-care costs and use of scarce acute care resources are important considerations in most countries, and they are an often unspoken factor in EOL decisions and the care of patients on life-support. A qualitative study of Canadian perspectives found resource allocation and its fair use and distribution to be the most ethically challenging issue for Canadian physicians (Rodrigue et al., 2013). For some health-care providers, it was an almost taboo subject: "[I] know resources influence the decision but we are not supposed to talk about that because nobody wants to think that we decide about one patient on the basis of not enough beds." The need for social debate about resource allocation is raised repeatedly. Nevertheless, the extent to which physicians perceive their ethical responsibilities in relation to resource allocation varies, from having an active role to being absent altogether (Rodrigue et al., 2013).

The principle of justice requires that vulnerable patients, such as brain-damaged patients, be treated equally and no differently than healthy individuals or patients suffering from other conditions (Laureys, 2005). The principle of justice also refers to equity, in that the decisions that are taken have to be fair to other patients and society. This is an issue that has not been extensively discussed (Wade, 2001). As put forth by Congedo and Zullo (2012):

> [i]s it equitable to allocate substantial but scare resources to someone who is unaware of his own situation? Which criteria of social justice should we apply locally if we want to make an equal distribution of resources amongst those who have a legitimate claim on them?

Accordingly, physicians and health-care professionals may have to consider the benefit that a treatment can bring to a patient as well as to other patients (Jonsen, Siegler, & Winslade, 1998). Several authors and commentators have argued that if a treatment is considered futile for a patient (i.e., that there is less than a 1% chance of physiological benefit), then it is not unethical to use otherwise unavailable resources for another patient that would directly benefit from them (Jonsen, Siegler, & Winslade, 1998). Medical futility is often defined as the situation in which a therapy that is hoped to benefit a patient's medical condition will predictably not do so on the basis of the best available evidence (Laureys, 2005). Caution is warranted regarding the notion of futility since diverse and conflicting understandings of this concept have been reported. For example, health-care professionals have been reported to vary not only on their definition of futility (Bernat, 2005), but also on the context in which they use it (e.g., clinical team versus family setting). Moreover, the family and the clinical team do not often agree as to what constitutes futile care. These differences in medical and societal practices concerning the distribution of resources for the long-term care of patients with DOC appear to shape ethical attitudes and clinical practice (Kuehlmeyer, 2014). Although wide agreement on such sensitive issues is unlikely to be achieved soon, institutions would benefit from having clearer policies to guide clinicians facing such difficult decisions.

Other challenges created by the management of scarce resources include situations in which patients are transferred from acute-care hospitals to long-term and rehabilitation centers because of financial or other pressures. The transfer of patients between institutions can affect patients insofar as the vision of health-care professionals (e.g., curative, palliative) may differ from one institution to another. In addition, recovery can take many months and long-term care facilities need to be tooled to identify patients who need additional services and resources (Fins, 2005a, b). Often, patients with DOC are cared for in the home-care setting, with relatives having to strain for financial support in addition to bearing the emotional and physical burden.

Conclusion

Both the clinical and neuroscience dimensions of DOC are complicated by vexing issues like resource allocation and high levels of diagnostic inaccuracies (at least for the VS/UWS). Other issues, like withdrawal of life-support, which had been considered "settled" by many in the medical, legal, and ethical communities, have resurfaced under the pressure of social groups and religious authorities as well as in light of scientific advances. Developments in scientific understanding of the MCS and the VS/UWS may gradually alter some assumptions about the level of awareness and the prognosis of these patients. These advances, which are tricky to interpret, and the hope and expectations they nourish in families and in the public, will need to be addressed concretely at the bedside. We identified several areas ripe for further interdisciplinary medical research on the ethical and social aspects of DOC. We suggest a need for a broad research and policy agenda that would shed more light on the scientific, medical, social, and ethical landscape of DOC.

Further research on diagnosis and prognosis

Develop fundamental and applied interdisciplinary research to increase the evidence base for diagnosis and prognosis. This implies sidestepping "therapeutic nihilism" and existing biases against this patient population to develop and fund research across different institutions (Racine, Rodrigue, et al., 2010).

Promoting ongoing clinical education

Develop and assess institutional and professional educational programs on clinical aspects of DOC and associated ethical challenges. This will become increasingly important with predictable changes to diagnoses and prognoses based on the use of new treatment strategies and new diagnostic tools (Racine, Rodrigue, et al., 2010).

Developing bottom-up research

Better understand the experience of health-care providers and family members. Too often, the experience of health-care professionals is unvoiced and is not fully considered in the treatment of chronically unresponsive patients (Racine, Rodrigue, et al., 2010).

Communication and public understanding

Better identify and characterize common challenges in matters of health-care communication and develop strategies to tackle potential miscommunications and sources of misunderstanding. To better prepare for difficult discussions with families, research is needed to help identify and characterize potential zones of tensions as well as approaches that can be employed by clinical teams and that could have a broader health policy application (Racine, Rodrigue, et al., 2010).

Shared decision-making

Develop tools and approaches to support shared decision-making and ensure respect for the patient and family members. Experiences with proxy decision-making and the interpretation of advance directives need to be gathered and shared to better understand the complexities of these situations and the different challenging aspects of this process (Racine, Rodrigue, et al., 2010).

Understanding prevalence, burden, and neuroepidemiology

Better understand the incidence of DOC as well as patient and family needs in matters of acute and long-term care. The burden of DOC is not well characterized, and better understanding the prevalence and medicosocial impact would help tailor acute interventions and long-term care needs and programs, as well as long-term support for families and caregivers (Racine, Rodrigue, et al., 2010).

Developing international collaboration and dialogue

Ensure greater consistency between different practice communities at local, national, and international levels in matters of care, terminology, and communication. Cross talk between different professional societies and interested parties is necessary to consolidate perspectives (Racine, Rodrigue, et al., 2010).

Acknowledgments

The writing of this chapter was made possible by an IRCM TD summer studentship (GW). ER benefits from the support of a career award from the Fonds de recherche du Québec – Santé (FRQ-S). Portions of this chapter have appeared in a previous publication: Racine E, Rodrigue C, Bernat J, Riopelle R, Shemie S. Observations on the Ethical and Social Aspects of Disorders of Consciousness. Can J Neurol Sci. 2010; 37: 758–768. We would like to thank Mr. Valentin Nguyen for editorial assistance in the preparation of this manuscript.

Notes

1 **Graham Wilson** is a summer student at the Neuroethics Research Unit, Institut de recherches cliniques de Montréal (IRCM), Montreal, Canada.
2 **Eric Racine** is Director of the Neuroethics Research Unit; associate IRCM research professor; associate director of scientific activities, academic affairs; associate research professor, Department of Medicine, University of Montreal; and adjunct professor, Department of Medicine (Division of Experimental Medicine) and Department of Neurology and Neurosurgery, McGill University.

References

Albrecht GL & Devlieger PJ. (1999). The disability paradox: high quality of life against all odds. *Soc Sci Med.* 48: 977–88.
American Academy of Neurology. (1989). Position of the American Academy of Neurology on certain aspects of the care and management of the persistent vegetative state patient. *Neurology.* 39(1): 125–126.
Andrews K. (1996). International Working Party on the Management of the Vegetative State: Summary Report. *Brain Injury.* 10: 797–806.
Andrews K, Murphy L, Munday R, & Littlewood C. (1996). Misdiagnosis of the vegetative state: retrospective study in a rehabilitation unit. *BMJ.* 313(7048): 13–16.
Asch DA, Faber-Langendoen K, Shea JA, et al. (1999). The sequence of withdrawing life-sustaining treatment from patients. *Am J Med.* 153–156.
Bacon D, Williams MA, & Gordon J. (2007). Position statement on laws and regulations concerning life-sustaining treatment, including artificial nutrition and hydration, for patients lacking decisionmaking capacity. *Neurology.* 68(14): 1097–1100.

Bardin JC, Fins JJ, Katz DI, et al. (2011). Dissociations between behavioural and functional magnetic resonance imaging-based evaluations of cognitive function after brain injury. *Brain.* 134(Pt 3): 769–782.

Bell TN. (1986). Nurses' attitudes in caring for the comatose head-injured patient. *J Neurosci Nurs.* 18(5): 279–289.

Bernat JL. (2004). Ethical aspects of determining and communicating prognosis in critical care. *Neurocrit Care.* 1: 107–117.

Bernat JL. (2005). Medical futility: Definition, determination, and disputes in critical care. *Neurocritical Care.* 2(2): 198–205.

Bernat JL. (2006). Chronic disorders of consciousness. *Lancet.* 367: 1181–1192.

Bernat JL & Rottenberg DA. (2007). Conscious awareness in PVS and MCS: the borderlands of Neurology. *Neurology.* 68: 885–886.

Bernat JL. (2009). Ethical issues in the treatment of severe brain injury. The impact of new technologies. Disorders of consciousness. *Ann N Y Acad Sci.* 1157: 117–130.

Boards of directors of the Canadian Healthcare Association, Canadian Medical Association, Canadian Nurses Association, Catholic Health Association of Canada. Joint statement on preventing and resolving ethical conflicts involving health care providers and persons receiving care. (1999). Retrieved from http://www.cna-nurses.ca/CNA/documents/pdf/publications/prevent_resolv_ethical_conflict_e.pdf

Boly M, Faymonville ME, Schnakers C, Peigneux P, Lambermont B, Phillips C, Lancellotti P, Luxen A, Lamy M, Moonen G, Maquet P, & Laureys, S. (2008). Perception of pain in the minimally conscious state with PET activation: an observational study. *Lancet Neurology.* 7: 1013–1020.

Brukamp K. (2012). Vegetative State? – A definition revisited. In Jox RJ, Kuehlmeyer K, Marckmann G, Racine E (Eds.). *Vegetative State – A Paradigmatic Problem of Modern Societies: Medical, Ethical, Legal and Social Perspectives on Chronic Disorders of Consciousness.* Münster: Lit Verlag: 7–18.

Bruno MA, Laureys S, & Demertzi A. (2013). Coma and disorders of consciousness. In Bernat JL, Beresford, R (Eds.). *Handbook of Clinical Neurology.* Netherlands: Elsevier: 201–211.

Buechler CM, Blostein PA, Koestner A, Hurt K, Schaars M, & McKernan J. (1998). Variation among trauma centers' calculation of Glasgow Coma Scale score: results of a national survey. *J Trauma.* 45(3): 429–432.

Canadian Medical Association. (1992). Advance directives for resuscitation and other life-saving or sustaining measures. *CMAJ.* 146(6): 1072A–B.

Canadian Medical Association. (2004). CMA Code of ethics. Retrieved from http://policy base.cma.ca/PolicyPDF/PD04–06.pdf

Chatelle C, Majerus S, Whyte J, Laureys S, & Schnakers C. (2012). A sensitive scale to assess nociceptive pain in patients with disorders of consciousness. *J Neurol Neurosurg Psychiatry.* 83: 1233–1237.

Childs NL, Mercer WN, & Childs HW. (1993). Accuracy of diagnosis of persistent vegetative state. *Neurology.* 43(8): 1465–1467.

Chwala-Schlegel N & Schabus N. (2012). Neuroscientific progress using EEG in disorders of consciousness research. In Jox RJ, Kuehlmeyer K, Marckmann G, Racine E (Eds.). *Vegetative State – A Paradigmatic Problem of Modern Societies: Medical, Ethical, Legal and Social Perspectives on Chronic Disorders of Consciousness.* Münster: Lit Verlag: 41–55.

Coleman MR, Davis MH, Rodd JM, et al. (2009). Towards the routine use of brain imaging to aid the clinical diagnosis of disorders of consciousness. *Brain.* 132: 2541–2552.

Coleman MR, Rodd JM, Davis MH, Johnsrude IS, Menon DK, Pickard JD, & Owen AM. (2007). Do vegetative patients retain aspects of language comprehension? Evidence from fMRI. *Brain*. 130: 2494–2507.

Congedo M, & Zullo S. (2012). Assistance for post-coma patients in vegetative state: two different models in Italian regional regulations considered from the local justice point of view. In Caplan A (Ed.). *Pragmatic Neuroethics*. Cambridge: MIT Press: 111–118.

Cook DJ, Guyatt GH, Jaeschke R, et al. (1995). Life support in the intensive care unit: a qualitative investigation of technological ventilation in anticipation of death in the intensive care unit. *N Engl J Med*. 349: 1123–1132.

Crossman J, Bankes M, Bhan A, & Crockard HA. (1998). The Glasgow Coma Score: reliable evidence? *Injury*. 29(6): 435–437.

Cruse D, Chennu S, Chatelle C, Bekinschtein TA, Fernández-Espejo D, et al. (2011). Bedside detection of awareness in the vegetative state. *Lancet*; 378(9809): 2088–2094.

Cruse D, Chennu S, Chatelle C, Fernández-Espejo D, Bekinschtein TA, et al. (2012). The relationship between aetiology and covert cognition in the minimally conscious state. *Neurology*. 78: 816–822.

Demertzi A, Ledoux D, Bruno MA, Vanhaudenhuyse A, Gosseries O, Soddu A, Schnakers C, Moonen G, & Laureys S. (2011). Attitudes towards end-of-life issues in disorders of consciousness: a European survey. *J Neurol*. 258: 1058–1065.

Demertzi A, Racine E, Bruno M-A, LeDoux D, Gosseries O, Vanhaudenhuyse A, Thonnard M, Soddu A, Moonen G, & Laureys S. (2013). Pain perception in disorders of consciousness: neuroscience, clinical care, and ethics in dialogue. *Neuroethics*. 6(1): 37–50.

Di HB, Yu SM, Weng XC, et al. (2007). Cerebral response to patient's own name in the vegetative and minimally conscious states. *Neurology*. 68: 895–899.

Estraneo A, Moretta P, Loreto V, Lanzillo B, Santoro L, & Trojano L. (2010). Late recovery after traumatic, anoxic, or hemorrhagic long-lasting vegetative state. *Neurology*. 75(3): 239–245.

Fernández-Espejo D, Bekinschtein T, Monti M, et al. (2011). Diffusion weighted imaging distinguishes the vegetative state from the minimally conscious state. *Neuroimage*. 54(1): 103–112.

Ferreira N. (2007). Latest legal and social developments in the euthanasia debate: bad moral consciences and political unrest. *Med Law*. 26: 387–407.

Fins JJ. (2005a). Clinical pragmatism and the care of brain damaged patients: toward a palliative neuroethics for disorders of consciousness. *Prog Brain Res*. 150: 565–582.

Fins JJ. (2005b). Rethinking disorders of consciousness: new research and its implications. *Hastings Cent Report*. 35: 22–24.

Fins JJ. (2010). Neuroethics, neuroimaging, and disorders of consciousness: promise or peril. *Transactions of the American Clinical and Climatological Association*. (122): 336–346.

Fins JJ, Illes J, Bernat JL, Hirsch J, Laureys S, & Murphy E. (2008). Neuroimaging and disorders of consciousness: envisioning an ethical research agenda. *American Journal of Bioethics*. 8(9): 3–12.

Fins JJ & Schiff ND. (2006). Shades of gray: new insights into the vegetative state. *Hastings Center Report*. 36: 8.

Gaccino JT, Zasler ND, Katz DI, Kelly JP, Rosenberg JH, & Filley CM. (1997). Development of practice guidelines for assessment and management of the vegetative and minimally conscious states. *J Head Trauma Rehabil*. 12(4): 79–89.

Ganz FD, Benbenishty J, Hersch M, Fischer A, Gurman G, & Sprung CL. (2006). The impact of regional culture on intensive care end of life decision making: an Israeli perspective from the ETHICUS study. *J Med Ethics*. 32(4): 196–199.

Gevers S. (2005). Withdrawing life support from patients in a persistent vegetative state: the law in the Netherlands. *Eur J Health Law.* 12: 347–355.

Giacino J, Kalmar K, & Whyte J. (2004). The JFK Coma Recovery Scale-Revised: measurement characteristics and diagnostic utility. *Arch Phys Med Rehabil.* 85(12): 2020–2029.

Gill-Thwaites H. (2006). Lotteries, loopholes and luck: misdiagnosis in the vegetative state patient. *Brain Inj.* 20(13–14): 1321–1328.

Gillick MR, Hesse K, & Mazzapica N. (1993). Medical technology at the end of life. What would physicians and nurses want for themselves? *Arch Intern Med.* (153): 2542–2547.

Godlovitch G, Mitchell I, & Doig CJ. (2005). Discontinuing life support in comatose patients: an example from Canadian case law. *CMAJ.* 172(9): 1172–1173.

Gofton TE, Chouinard PA, Young GB, et al. (2009). Functional MRI study of the primary somatosensory cortex in comatose survivors of cardiac arrest. *Exp Neurol.* 217(2): 320–327.

Gosseries O, Bruno MA, Chatelle C, Vanhaudenhuyse A, Schnakers C, Soddu A, et al. (2004). Disorders of consciousness: what's in a name? *NeuroRehabilitation.* 19(4): 293–298.

Grubb A, Walsh P, Lambe N, Murrells T, & Robinson S. (1996). Survey of British clinicians' views on management of patients in persistent vegetative state. *Lancet.* 348(9019): 35–40.

Hirschberg R & Giacino JT. (2011). The vegetative and minimally conscious states: diagnosis, prognosis and treatment. *Neurol Clin.* 29: 773–786.

Hopkin M. (2006). "Vegetative" patient shows signs of conscious thought. *Nature.* 443: 132–133.

Huber B & Kuehlmeyer K. (2012). Perspectives of family caregivers on the vegetative state. In Jox RJ, Kuehlmeyer K, Marckmann G, Racine E (Eds.). *Vegetative State – A Paradigmatic Problem of Modern Societies: Medical, Ethical, Legal and Social Perspectives on Chronic Disorders of Consciousness.* Münster: Lit Verlag: 97–109.

Huisman TA, Schwamm LH, Schaefer PW, et al. (2004). Diffusion tensor imaging as potential biomarker of white matter injury in diffuse axonal injury. *AJNR Am J Neuroradiol.* 25(3): 370–376.

Hurst SA, Perrier A, Pegoraro R, Reiter-Theil S, Forde R, Slowther AM, Garrett-Mayer E, & Danis M. (2007). Ethical difficulties in clinical practice: experiences of European doctors. *J Med Ethics* 33(1): 51–57.

Jeffery D. (2005). *Patient-Centred Ethics and Communication at the End of Life.* Oxford: Radcliffe Publishing.

Jennett B. (1976). Editorial: Recourse allocation for the severely brain damaged. *Arch Neurol.* 33: 595–597.

John Paul II. (2004). Address of John Paul II to the participants in the International Congress on "Life-sustaining treatments and vegetative state: Scientific advances and ethical dilemmas." Vatican. Retrieved from http://www.vatican.va/holy_father/john_paul_ii/speeches/2004/march/documents/hf_jp-ii_spe_20040320_congressfiamc_en.html

Jonsen AR, Siegler M, & Winslade WT. (1998). *Clinical Ethics: A Practical Approach to Ethical Decisions in Clinical Medicine.* 4th ed. New York: McGraw Hill.

Jox R, Bernat J, Laureys S, & Racine E. (2012). Disorders of consciousness: responding to requests for novel diagnostic and therapeutic interventions. *Lancet Neurol.* 11: 732–738.

Jox RJ, Kuehlmeyer K, Marckmann G, & Racine E. (2012). Introduction. In Jox RJ, Kuehlmeyer K, Marckmann G, Racine E (Eds.). *Vegetative State – A Paradigmatic Problem of Modern Societies: Medical, Ethical, Legal and Social Perspectives on Chronic Disorders of Consciousness.* Münster: Lit Verlag: 1–3.

Keenan SP, Busche KD, Chen LM, et al. (1998). Withdrawal and withholding of life support in the intensive care unit: a comparison of teaching and community hospitals. The Southwestern Ontario Clinical Care Research Network. *Critical Care Med.* 26: 245–251.

Kuehlmeyer K, Borasio GD, & Jox R. (2012). How family caregivers' medical and moral assumptions influence decision making for patients in the vegetative state: a qualitative study. *J Med Ethics*. 38: 332–337.

Kuehlmeyer K, Klingler C, Racine E, & Jox RJ. (2013). Single case reports on late recovery from chronic disorders of consciousness: a systematic review and ethical appraisal. *Bioethics Forum*. 6(4): 137–149.

Kuehlmeyer K, Palmour N, Riopelle RJ, Bernat JL, Jox RJ, & Racine E. (2014). Physicians' attitudes toward medical and ethical challenges for patients in the vegetative state: comparing Canadian and German perspectives in a vignette survey. *BMC Neurology*. 14:119.

Kuehlmeyer K, Racine E, Palmour N, Hoster E, Borasio GD, & Jox RJ. (2012). Diagnostic and ethical challenges in disorders of consciousness and locked-in syndrome: a survey of German neurologists. *J Neurol*. 10: 2076–2089.

Lanzerath D, Honnefelder L, & Feeser U. (1998). Nationaler Bericht der europäischen Befragung: "Doctors' views on the management of patients in persistent vegetative state (PVS)" im Rahmen des Forschungsprojekts "The moral and legal issues surrounding the treatment and health care of patients in persistent vegetative state." *Ethik in der Medizin*. 10: 152–180.

Laureys S. (2007). Eyes open, brain shut. *Scientific American*. May: 32–37.

Laureys S. (2005). Science and society: death, unconsciousness and the brain. *Nat Rev Neurosci*. 6(11): 899–909.

Laureys S, Celesia GG, Cohadon F, et al. (2010). Unresponsive wakefulness syndrome: a new name for the vegetative state or apallic syndrome. *BMC Med*. 8: 68.

Laureys S, Faymonville ME, Peigneux P, et al. (2002). Cortical processing of noxious somatosensory stimuli in the persistent vegetative state. *NeuroImage*. 17: 732–741.

Laureys S, Owen AM, & Schiff ND. (2004). Brain function in coma, vegetative state and related disorders. *Lancet Neurol*. 3: 537–546.

Laureys S, Perrin F, Faymonville ME, et al. (2004). Cerebral processing in the minimally conscious state. *Neurology*. 63: 916–918.

Laureys S, Perrin F, Schnakers C, Boly M, & Majerus S. (2005). Residual cognitive function in comatose, vegetative and minimally conscious states. *Curr Opin Neurology*. 18: 726–733.

Lennard-Jones JE. (2000). Ethical and legal aspects of clinical hydration and nutritional support. *BJU Int*. 85(4): 398–403.

Luaute J, Maucort-Boulch D, Tell L, et al. (2010). Long term outcomes of chronic minimally conscious and vegetative states. *Neurology*. 75(3): 246–252.

Lulé D, Noirhomme Q, Kleih SC, et al. (2013). Probing command following in patients with disorders of consciousness using a brain-computer interface. *Clin Neurophysiol*. 124: 101–106.

Macdonald ME, Liben S, Carnevale FA, & Cohen SR. (2008). Signs of life and signs of death: brain death and other mixed messages at the end of life. J Child Health Care. 12(2): 92–105.

Machado C, Rodriguez R, Carballo M, Perez J, & Korein J. (2009). Results of proton MRS studies in PVS and MCS patients. *Can J Neurol Sci*. 36(3): 365–369.

Majerus S, Gill-Thwaites H, Andrews K, & Laureys S. (2005). Behavioural evaluation of consciousness in severe brain damage. In Laureys S (Ed.) *Progress in Brain Research*. Vol. 150 DOI: 10.1016/S0079-6123(05)50028-1.

Marcin JP, Pretzlaff RK, Pollack MM, et al. (1999). Certainty and morality prediction in critically ill children. *J Med Ethics*. (30): 304–307.

McCann A, Stowe J, Delargy M, & Carroll A. (2012). Uncovering hidden awareness-using the Sensory Modality Assessment and Rehabilitation Technique (SMART) to reduce potential misdiagnosis. In Jox RJ, Kuehlmeyer K, Marckmann G, Racine E (Eds.). *Vegetative State – A Paradigmatic Problem of Modern Societies: Medical, Ethical, Legal and Social Perspectives on Chronic Disorders of Consciousness.* Münster: Lit Verlag: 19–37.

Miller FG & Fins JJ. (2006). Protecting human subjects in brain research: a pragmatic perspective. In Illes J (Ed.). *Neuroethics: Defining the Issues in Theory, Practice, and Policy.* Oxford: Oxford University Press: 123–140.

Montagnino BA & Ethier AM. (2007). The experiences of pediatric nurses caring for children in a persistent vegetative state. *Pediatr Crit Care Med.* 8(5): 440–446.

Monti MM, Pickard JD, & Owen AM. (2012). Visual cognition in disorders of consciousness: from V1 to top-down attention. *Hum Brain Mapp.* 34(6): 1245–1253.

Monti MM, Vanhaudenhuyse A, Coleman MR, et al. (2010). Willful modulation of brain activity in disorders of consciousness. *N Engl J Med.* 362(7): 579–589.

Multi-Society Task Force on PVS. (1994). Medical aspects of the persistent vegetative state (2). *N Engl J Med.* 330(22): 1572–1579.

Nizzi MC, Demertzi A, Gosseries O, et al. (2012). From arm-chair to wheel-chair: how patients with a locked-in syndrome integrate bodily changes in experienced identity. *Concious Cogn.* 21: 431–437.

Overgaard M & Overgaard R. (2011). Measurements of consciousness in the vegetative state. *Lancet.* 378: 2052–2054.

Owen AM. (2013). Detecting consciousness: a unique role for neuroimaging. *Annu Rev Psychol.* 64: 109–133.

Owen AM & Coleman MR. (2008). Functional neuroimaging of the vegetative state. *Nat Rev Neurosi.* 9: 235–243.

Owen AM, Coleman MR, Boly M, Davis MH, Laureys S, & Pickard JD. (2006). Detecting awareness in the vegetative state. *Science.* 313(5792): 1402.

Payne K, Taylor RM, Stocking C, & Sachs GA. (1996). Physicians' attitudes about the care of patients in the persistent vegetative state: a national survey. *Ann Intern Med.* 125(2): 104–110.

Pence GE. (2004). Comas: Karen Quinlan and Nancy Cruzan. In Pence GE (Ed.). *Classic Cases on Medical Ethics.* Boston: McGraw-Hill: 29–57.

Perry JE, Churchill LR, & Kirshner HS. (2005). The Terri Schiavo case: legal, ethical, and medical perspectives. *Ann Intern Med.* 143(10): 744–748.

Phipps E & Whyte J. (1999). Medical decision-making with persons who are minimally conscious: a commentary. *Am J Phys Med Rehabil.* 78(1): 77–82.

Plum F & Posner JB. (1983). *The Diagnosis of Stupor and Coma.* Philadelphia: F.A Davis.

Pontifical Academy for Life and the World Federation of Catholic Medical Associations. Joint statement on the vegetative state. International Congress on "Life sustaining treatments and vegetative state: Scientific advances and ethical dilemmas"; March 10–17, 2004; Rome. Retrieved from http://www.vatican.va/roman_curia/pontifical_academies/acdlife/documents/rc_pont-acd_life_doc_20040320_jointstatement-veget-state_en.html

Post MW, de Witt LP, van Asbeck FW, et al. (1998). Predictors of health status and life satisfaction in spinal cord injury. *Arch Phys Med Rehabil.* 79: 395–401.

Powner DJ, Hernandez M, & Rives TE. (2004). Variability among hospital policies for determining brain death in adults. *Crit Care Med.* 32(6): 1284–1288.

Prendergast TJ, Claessens MT, & Luce JM. (1998). A national survey of end-of-life care for critically ill patients. *Am J Respir Crit Care Med.* 158: 1163–1167.

Racine E. (2010). Communication of prognosis in disorders of consciousness and severe brain injury: a closer look at paradoxical discourses in the clinical and public domains. In Caplan A (Ed.). *Pragmatic Neuroethics.* Cambridge: MIT Press: 161–178.

Racine E. (2013). Pragmatic neuroethics: the social aspects of ethics in disorders of consciousness. In Bernat JL, Beresford, R (Eds.). *Handbook of Clinical Neurology*. Netherlands: Elsevier: 366–369.

Racine E, Amaram R, Seidler M, Karczewska M, & Illes J. (2008). Media coverage of the persistent vegetative state and end-of-life decision-making. *Neurology*. 71(13): 1027–1032.

Racine E, Bar-Ilan O, & Illes J. (2006). Brain imaging: a decade of coverage in the print media. *Sci Commun*. 28: 122–142.

Racine E & Bell E. (2008). Clinical and public translation of neuroimaging research in disorders of consciousness challenges current diagnostic and public understanding paradigms. *Am J Bioeth*. 8(9): 13–15.

Racine E, Dion MJ, Wijman CA, Illes J, & Lansberg MG. (2009). Profiles of neurological outcome prediction among intensivists. *Neurocrit Care*. 11(3): 345–352.

Racine E, Lansberg MG, Dion M-J, et al. (2007). A qualitative study of prognostication and end-of-life decision making in critically-ill neurological patients. International Conference in Clinical Ethics, Toronto.

Racine E, Rodrigue C, Bernat J, Riopelle R, & Shemie S. (2010). Observations on the ethical and social aspects of disorders of consciousness. *Can J Neurol Sci*. 37: 758–768.

Racine E & Shevell MI. (2009). Ethics in neonatal neurology: when is enough, enough? *Pediatr Neurol*. 40(3): 147–155.

Racine E, Waldman S, Rosenberg J, & Illes J. (2010). Contemporary neuroscience in the media. *Soc Sci Med*. 71: 725–733.

Randolph AG, Zollo MB, Wigton RS, et al. (1997). Factors explaining variability among caregivers in the intent to restrict life-support interventions in a pediatric intensive care unit. *Crit Care Med*. 25: 435–439.

Rebagliato M, Cuttini M, Broggin L, et al. (2000). Neonatal end-of-life decision making: physicians' attitudes and relationship with self reported practices in 10 European countries. *JAMA*. 284(19): 2451–2459.

Rocker GM, Cook DJ, & Shemie SD. (2006). Practice variation in end of life care in the ICU: implications for patients with severe brain injury. *Can J Anaesth*. 53: 814–819.

Rodrigue C, Riopelle RJ, Bernat JL, & Racine E. (2013). How Contextual and Relational Aspects Shape the Perspective of Healthcare Providers on Decision Making for Patients With Disorders of Consciousness: A Qualitative Interview Study. *Narrative Inquiry in Bioethics*. 3: 261–273.

Schiff ND, Giacino JT, Kalmar K, et al. (2007). Behavioural improvements with thalamic stimulation after severe traumatic brain injury. *Nature*. 448(7153): 600–603.

Schiff ND, Rodriguez-Moreno D, Kamal A, et al. (2005). fMRI reveals large-scale network activation in minimally conscious patients. *Neurology*. 64: 514–523.

Schnakers C, Vanhaudenhuyse A, Giacino J, et al. (2009). Diagnostic accuracy of the vegetative and minimally conscious state: clinical consensus versus standardized neurobehavioral assessment. BMC Neurol. 9: 35.

Shanteau J & Linin K. (1990). Subjective meaning of terms used in organ donation: analysis of word associations. In Shanteau J, Harris, R (Eds.). *Organ Donation and Transplantation: Psychological and Behavioral Factors*. Washington: American Psychological Association: 37–49.

Shiel A, Gelling L, Wilson B, Coleman M, & Pickard JD. (2004). Difficulties in diagnosing the vegetative state. *Br J Neurosurg*. 18(1): 5–7.

Sim J. (1997). Ethical issues in the management of persistent vegetative state. *Physiother Res Int*. 2(2): 7–11.

Siminoff LA, Burant C, & Youngner SJ. (2004). Death and organ procurement: public beliefs and attitudes. *Kennedy Inst Ethics J.* 14(3): 217–234.

Siminoff LA, Mercer MB, & Arnold R. (2003). Families' understanding of brain death. *Prog Transplant.* 13(3): 218–224.

Singer PA, Robertson G, & Roy DJ. (1996). Bioethics for clinicians: 6. Advance care planning. *CMAJ.* 155(12): 1689–1692.

Sorger B, Reithler J, Dahman B, et al. (2012). A real-time fMRI based spelling device immediately enabling robust motor-independent communication. *Curr Biol.* 22: 1333–1338.

Spinney L. (2004). Blink and you live. The Guardian. April 15. Retrieved from http://www.gaurdian.co.uk/education/2004/apr/15/research.highereducation/print

Sprung CL, Cohen SL, Sjokvist, et al. (2003). End-of-life practices in European intensive care units: the Ethicus Study. *JAMA.* 290: 790–797.

Thompson T, Barbour R, & Scwartz L. (2003). Adherence to advance directives in critical care decision making: a vignette study. *Br Med J.* 327: 1–7.

Tomlinson T. (1990). Misunderstanding death on a respirator. *Bioethics.* 4(3): 253–264.

Tshibanda L, Vanhaudenhuyse A, Galanaud D, Boly M, Laureys S, & Puybasset L. (2009). Magnetic resonance spectroscopy and diffusion tensor imaging in coma survivors: promises and pitfalls. *Prog Brain Res.* 177: 215–229.

Voss HU, Uluc AM, Dyke JP, et al. (2006). Possible axonal regrowth in late recovery from the minimally conscious state. *J Clin Invest.* 116(7): 2005–2011.

Wade DT. (2001). Ethical issues in diagnosis and management of patients in the permanent vegetative state. *BMJ.* 322(7282): 352–354.

Wijdicks EF & Wijdicks CA. (2006). The portrayal of coma in contemporary motion pictures. *Neurology.* 66(9): 1300–1303.

Wijdicks EF & Wijdicks MF. (2006). Coverage of coma in headlines of US newspapers from 2001 through 2005. *Mayo Clin Proc.* 81(10): 1332–1336.

Wilkinson DJ, Kahane G, Horne M, & Savulescu J. (2009). Functional neuroimaging and withdrawal of life-sustaining treatment from vegetative patients. *J Med Ethics.* 35(8): 508–511.

Wilson FC, et al. (2007). Vegetative and minimally conscious state(s) survey: attitudes of clinical neuropsychologists and speech and language therapists. *Disability and Rehabilitation.* 29(22): 1751–1756.

Young B, Blume W, & Lynch A. (1989). Brain death and the persistent vegetative state: similarities and contrasts. *Can J Neurol Sci.* 16(4): 388–393.

Youngner SJ, Landefeld CS, Coulton CJ, Juknialis BW, & Leary M. (1989). Brain death and organ retrieval. A cross-sectional survey of knowledge and concepts among health professionals. *JAMA.* 261(15): 2205–2210.

Yuan W, Holland SK, Schmithorst VJ, et al. (2007). Diffusion tensor MR imaging reveals persistent white matter alteration after traumatic brain injury experienced during early childhood. *AJNR Am J Neuroradiol.* 28(10): 1919–1925.

Zeman A. (1997). Persistent vegetative state. *Lancet.* 350(9080): 795–799.

8 Conclusion and future perspectives

Camille Chatelle[1] and Steven Laureys[2]

Abbreviations

DOC   disorders of consciousness
MCS   minimally conscious state
MCS★   nonbehavioral MCS
UWS   unresponsive wakefulness syndrome
VS   vegetative state

Over the years, the increasing number of patients who survive severe brain damage but remain poorly responsive and noncommunicative at the bedside for months or years has led to a striking need to better characterize, understand, and manage this population.

The "vegetative state" (VS) was first defined by Jennett and Plum in 1972 to describe patients who show no sign of consciousness at the bedside but who show a preservation of autonomic functions (e.g., cardiovascular regulation, thermoregulation) and arousal (i.e., eyes open). Recently, Laureys and colleagues suggested replacing the term "vegetative" with "unresponsive wakefulness syndrome" (UWS) in order to avoid the negative connotations associated with the previous term and to better describe the behavioral pattern observed in this population (Laureys et al., 2010). In 2002, a new clinical entity was introduced by the Aspen Group to account for patients who did not fully recover consciousness but who retained fluctuating but consistent signs of awareness at the bedside and therefore could not be considered as unresponsive to their environment. They called this the "minimally conscious state" (MCS, Giacino et al., 2002). More recently, it has been suggested that this clinical entity actually encompasses a broad, heterogeneous population of patients with different cognitive abilities, and therefore it could be possible to subcategorize it into "MCS minus" and "MCS plus" depending on the patient's degree of language preservation (Bruno et al., 2012; Bruno, Vanhaudenhuyse, Thibaut, Moonen, & Laureys, 2011).

The definitions of the clinical entities lying between deep coma and full recovery of consciousness have evolved with our understanding of severely brain-injured patients. A significant amount of research has attempted to characterize residual cognitive processing using different methods, some of which create a real uneasiness in the clinical field. In 2008, a study reported brain response to noxious stimuli in patients in a MCS similar to that which could be observed in healthy controls, suggesting that these patients, even though noncommunicative, could have the capacity to process painful stimulation and, therefore, should be assessed and treated when appropriate (Boly et al., 2008). One year later, a study showed that about 41% of patients with a severe brain injury may be misdiagnosed by the clinical team if standardized tools are not used to assess the patient at the bedside (Schnakers et al., 2009). Finally, several reports of patients thought to be unconscious at the bedside who are able to follow commands by modulating their brain activity multiplied the questions surrounding diagnostic accuracy in this population (Owen et al., 2006).

As illustrated by these few examples, recent findings have raised important ethical and medical concerns regarding care management of brain-injured patients with disorders of consciousness (DOC). The challenge of assessing pain and managing analgesic treatment with limited or no subjective report has highlighted the need for a better understanding of patients' pain processing and standardized validated tools to assess these patients.

In this book, we first reported on current knowledge of pain processing in humans. We highlighted the difficulty of inferring pain processing from current studies as no nociceptive-specific cortical area has yet been clearly described. However, if it makes findings from DOC more difficult to interpret, it does not erase the fact that some patients retain the ability to perceive painful stimulation and should therefore be treated when appropriate. Additionally, though we still know very little about acute pain processing in DOC, we do not even know anything about chronic pain in these patients. Future studies should try to better understand chronic and neuropathic pain in a communicative population in order to further investigate whether the brain lesions leading to DOC could also lead to unrecognized states of neuropathic pain (see Chapter 2).

As behavioral assessments remain the "gold standard" for assessing pain and communication, we explored some keys to objectively assessing patients with DOC using standardized or individualized tools. The Nociception Coma Scale Revised (Chatelle, Majerus, Whyte, Laureys, & Schnakers, 2012; Schnakers et al., 2010) has been validated to assess acute pain in noncommunicative brain-injured patients and can be used to manage pain treatment in DOC (see Chapter 3). However, future studies need to investigate the clinical usability of the scale within short- and long-term settings, to see whether it is useful to manage pain during potentially painful acts of care. Additionally, the question of how to detect and manage chronic pain in these patients still needs to be investigated. More research in this field will support the development of guidelines regarding the management of pain in DOC, helping clinicians to avoid situations in which patients remain untreated, in addition to guidelines for adapting antalgic treatment, improving the comfort and outcome in this population.

In the context of clinical management of DOC, assessing consciousness and communication is a key to providing appropriate treatment and rehabilitation. Standardized tools such as the Coma Recovery Scale-Revised (Giacino, Kalmar, & Whyte, 2004), in combination with individually tailored assessment protocols such as the Quantitative Individualized Behavioral Assessment, can help monitor a patient's recovery and improve the diagnosis (see Chapter 4).

Although behavioral assessment remains the "gold standard" for assessing consciousness and communication, it is highly motor-dependent and it may not be completely reliable with patient suffering severe motor impairment. For this reason, we also discussed the current work on the development of paraclinical tools to detect command-following and to communicate with severely brain-injured patients. Active paradigms have been developed using cortically-based techniques (e.g., functional magnetic resonance imaging, electroencephalography) and non-cortically-based techniques (e.g., electromyography, pupil dilation, breath control) to detect covert cognition in patients with DOC. Although studies highlight the potential of these methods, they are usually not user-friendly and a high rate of false negatives is reported (i.e., patients showing command-following at the bedside who could not be detected with the method). Therefore, additional studies are needed so that tools that are easier to use and more sensitive can be developed and so that clinicians can better interpret and understand positive findings. If they are available, paraclinical assessments should, at this point, only be considered in the case of absence of consciousness or communication at the bedside and/or positive findings, and behavioral assessment will always prevail in case of negative findings (see Chapter 5).

Reports on patients who are unresponsive at the bedside showing the ability to modulate their brain activity in response to commands raised a new discussion on the clinical definition of these cases. To answer this question, the term "nonbehavioral MCS" (abbreviated as MCS*, Gosseries, Zasler, & Laureys, 2014) has been proposed to describe these patients. In the future, we will need to better characterize this new clinical entity and define future steps for care and rehabilitation in those patients (Bruno et al., 2011).

Paraclinical assessments could also help us avoid diagnosing a patient as VS/UWS or MCS despite their suffering from locked-in syndrome. In this case, as the patient retains full cognitive capacities, establishing communication will be a major step as it can improve the quality of life as well as the management of care in this population. Future studies will need to work on reliable tools to be used in completely paralyzed patients (see Chapter 6).

Last but not least, the implementation of these technologies in clinical settings will necessitate ethical and scientific discussions about how to adapt the definition of competency for patients communicating with a brain-computer interface (binary or spelling communication code) in order to allow them to be part of the decision-making process about their own rehabilitation, treatment, and end-of-life decisions, and also to enable them to reintegrate into the community (Bendtsen, 2013, see Chapter 7).

Notes

1 **Camille Chatelle** is a postdoctoral research fellow at the Neurorehabilitation Lab at the Spaulding Rehabilitation Hospital, Harvard Medical School. She is also working as a postdoctoral researcher at the Laboratory for NeuroImaging of Coma and Consciousness at Massachusetts General Hospital, Harvard Medical School.
2 **Steven Laureys** leads the Coma Science Group at the Cyclotron Research Center and Department of Neurology, Sart Tilman Liège University Hospital, Belgium. He is Clinical Professor and Research Director at the Belgian National Fund of Scientific Research (FNRS).

References

Bendtsen, K. (2013). Communicating with the minimally conscious: ethical implications in end-of-life care. *AJOB Neuroscience, 4*(1), 46–51.

Boly, M., Faymonville, M. E., Schnakers, C., Peigneux, P., Lambermont, B., Phillips, C., . . . Laureys, S. (2008). Perception of pain in the minimally conscious state with PET activation: an observational study. *The Lancet Neurology, 7*(11), 1013–1020.

Bruno, M. A., Majerus, S., Boly, M., Vanhaudenhuyse, A., Schnakers, C., Gosseries, O., . . . Laureys, S. (2012). Functional neuroanatomy underlying the clinical subcategorization of minimally conscious state patients. *J Neurol, 259*(6), 1087–1098.

Bruno, M. A., Vanhaudenhuyse, A., Thibaut, A., Moonen, G., & Laureys, S. (2011). From unresponsive wakefulness to minimally conscious PLUS and functional locked-in syndromes: recent advances in our understanding of disorders of consciousness. *J Neurol, 258*(7), 1373–1384.

Chatelle, C., Majerus, S., Whyte, J., Laureys, S., & Schnakers, C. (2012). A sensitive scale to assess nociceptive pain in patients with disorders of consciousness. *J Neurol Neurosurg Psychiatry, 83*(12), 1233–1237.

Giacino, J., Ashwal, S., Childs, N., Cranford, R., Jennett, B., Katz, D., . . . Zafonte, R. (2002). The minimally conscious state: Definition and diagnostic criteria. *Neurology, 58*(3), 349–353.

Giacino, J., Kalmar, K., & Whyte, J. (2004). The JFK Coma Recovery Scale-Revised: measurement characteristics and diagnostic utility. *Arch Phys Med Rehabil, 85*(12), 2020–2029.

Gosseries, O., Zasler, N. D., & Laureys, S. (2014). Recent advances in disorders of consciousness: focus on the diagnosis. *Brain Inj, 28*(9), 1141–1150.

Jennett, B., & Plum, F. (1972). Persistent vegetative state after brain damage. A syndrome in search of a name. *Lancet, 1*, 734–737.

Laureys, S., Celesia, G. G., Cohadon, F., Lavrijsen, J., Leon-Carrion, J., Sannita, W. G., . . . Dolce, G. (2010). Unresponsive wakefulness syndrome: a new name for the vegetative state or apallic syndrome. *BMC Med, 8*, 68.

Owen, A. M., Coleman, M. R., Boly, M., Davis, M. H., Laureys, S., & Pickard, J. D. (2006). Detecting awareness in the vegetative state. *Science, 313*(5792), 1402.

Schnakers, C., Chatelle, C., Vanhaudenhuyse, A., Majerus, S., Ledoux, D., Boly, M., . . . Laureys, S. (2010). The Nociception Coma Scale: a new tool to assess nociception in disorders of consciousness. *Pain, 148*(2), 215–219.

Schnakers, C., Vanhaudenhuyse, A., Giacino, J., Ventura, M., Boly, M., Majerus, S., . . . Laureys, S. (2009). Diagnostic accuracy of the vegetative and minimally conscious state: clinical consensus versus standardized neurobehavioral assessment. *BMC Neurology, 9*(1), 35.

Index